# RESPIRATORY CARE CALCULATIONS

## Second Edition

**David W. Chang, Ed.D., R.R.T.**

Director, Professor
Respiratory Therapy Program
Columbus State University
Columbus, Georgia

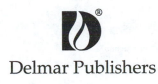

Delmar Publishers

*an International Thomson Publishing company* I(T)P®

Albany • Bonn • Boston • Cincinnati • Detroit • London • Madrid
Melbourne • Mexico City • New York • Pacific Grove • Paris • San Francisco
Singapore • Tokyo • Toronto • Washington

# NOTICE TO THE READER

Cover Design: Brucie Rosch

**Delmar Staff**
Publisher: Susan Simpfenderfer
Acquisitions Editor: Dawn Gerrain
Developmental Editor: Deb Flis
Marketing Manager: Darryl Caron
Marketing Coordinator: Nina Lontrato
Production Manager: Linda Helfrich
Production Coordinator: John Mickelbank
Editorial Assistant: Donna Leto
Team Assistant: Sandra Bruce

COPYRIGHT © 1999
By Delmar Publishers Inc.
*An International Thomson Publishing Company* I(T)P®

The ITP logo is a trademark under license
Printed in Canada

For more information, contact:

**JOIN US ON THE WEB: www.DelmarAlliedHealth.com**

*Your Information Resource!*
- What's New from Delmar • Health Science News Headlines
- Web Links to Many Related Sites
- Instructor Forum/Teaching Tips • Give Us Your Feedback
- Online Companions™
- Complete Allied Health Catalog • Software/Media Demos
- And much more!

**Delmar Online** To access a wide variety of Delmar products and services on the World Wide Web, point your browser to: **http://www.delmar.com/delmar.html**

A service of I(T)P®

**Delmar Publishers Inc.**
3 Columbia Circle, Box 15015
Albany, New York 12212-5015

**International Thomson Publishing Europe**
Berkshire House
168-173 High Holborn
London, WC1V 7AA
England

**Nelson ITP, Australia**
102 Dodds Street
South Melbourne
Victoria, 3205 Australia

**Nelson Canada**
1120 Birchmont Road
Scarborough, Ontario
M1K 5G4, Canada

**International Thomson Publishing France**
Tour Maine-Montparnasse
33 Avenue du Maine
75755 Paris Cedex 15, France

**International Thomson Editores**
Seneca 53
Colonia Polanco
11560 Mexico D F Mexico

**International Thomson Publishing GmbH**
Königswinterer Strasbe 418
53227 Bonn
Germany

**International Thomson Publishing Asia**
60 Albert Stree #15-01
Albert Complex
Singapore 189969

**International Thomson Publishing Japan**
Hirakawa-cho Kyowa Building, 3F
2-2-1 Hirakawa-cho, Chiyoda-ku,
Tokyo 102, Japan

**ITE Spain/Paraninfo**
Calle Magallanes, 25
28015-Madrid, Spain

1 2 3 4 5 6 7 8 9 XXX 03 02 01 00 99 98

**Library of Congress Cataloging-in Publication Data**
Chang, David W.
    Respiratory care calculations / David W. Chang. — 2nd ed.
        p.    cm.
    Includes bibliographical references and index.
    ISBN: 0-7668-0517-4
    1. Respiratory therapy—Mathematics.  2. Pulmonary function tests—Mathematics.    I. Title
    [DNLM: 1. Respiratory Physiology—methods programmed instruction.
    2. Monitoring, Physiologic—methods programmed instruction.
    3. Mathematics programmed instruction.    WF 18.2  C456r  1998]
    RC735.I5C47      1998
    612.2'0048—dc21
    DNLM/DLC
    for Library of Congress                                          98-43498
                                                                          CIP

# Contents

**Listing by Subject Areas**  v

**Preface**  vii

**Acknowledgments**  viii

*Section 1*  **Review of Basic Math Functions**  1
Review of Basic Math Functions  3

*Section 2*  **Respiratory Care Calculations**  7

1  Airway Resistance: Estimated ($R_{aw}$)  9
2  Alveolar–Arterial Oxygen Tension Gradient $P(A-a)O_2$  11
3  Alveolar Oxygen Tension ($P_AO_2$)  14
4  Anion Gap  16
5  Arterial/Alveolar Oxygen Tension ($a/A$) Ratio  18
6  Arterial–Mixed Venous Oxygen Content Difference $[C(a-\bar{v})O_2]$  20
7  ATPS to BTPS  23
8  Bicarbonate Corrections of Base Deficit  25
9  Body Surface Area  27
10  Cardiac Index ($CI$)  29
11  Cardiac Output ($CO$): Fick's Estimated Method  32
12  Compliance: Dynamic ($C_{dyn}$)  35
13  Compliance: Static ($C_{st}$)  38
14  Compliance: Total ($C_T$)  41
15  Corrected Tidal Volume ($V_T$)  43
16  Correction Factor  45
17  Dalton's Law of Partial Pressure  49
18  Deadspace to Tidal Volume Ratio ($V_D/V_T$)  51
19  Density ($D$) of Gases  54
20  Dosage Calculation: Intravenous Solution Infusion Dosage  57
21  Dosage Calculation: Intravenous Solution Infusion Rate  60
22  Dosage Calculation: Percent (%) Solutions  63
23  Dosage Calculation: Unit Dose  67
24  Dosage Estimated for Children: Young's Rule  72
25  Dosage Estimation for Infants and Children: Clark's Rule  74
26  Dosage Estimation for Infants and Children: Fried's Rule  76
27  Elastance ($E$)  78
28  Endotracheal Tube Size for Children  80
29  Fick's Law of Diffusion  83
30  $F_IO_2$ from Two Gas Sources  86
31  $F_IO_2$ Needed for a Desired $P_aO_2$  89
32  $F_IO_2$ Needed for a Desired $P_aO_2$ (COPD Patients)  91
33  Flow Rate in Mechanical Ventilation  93
34  Forced Vital Capacity Tracing (FEV$_t$ and FEV$_{t\%}$)  95
35  Forced Vital Capacity Tracing (FEF$_{200\text{-}1200}$)  102
36  Forced Vital Capacity Tracing (FEF$_{25\text{-}75\%}$)  110
37  Gas Law Equations  120
38  Gas Volume Corrections  123
39  Graham's Law of Diffusion Coefficient  126
40  Helium/Oxygen (He/O$_2$) Flow Rate Conversion  128
41  Humidity Deficit  130
42  I:E Ratio  132
43  Law of LaPlace  138
44  Lung Volumes and Capacities  140
45  Mean Airway Pressure ($MAWP$)  147
46  Mean Arterial Pressure ($MAP$)  151
47  Metric Conversion: Length  153
48  Metric Conversion: Volume  156
49  Metric Conversion: Weight  159
50  Minute Ventilation during IMV  162
51  Minute Ventilation: Expired and Alveolar  164
52  Oxygen: Air (O$_2$:Air) Entrainment Ratio  168
53  Oxygen Consumption ($\dot{V}O_2$) and Index ($\dot{V}O_2$ Index)  172
54  Oxygen Content: Arterial ($C_aO_2$)  176
55  Oxygen Content: End-Capillary ($C_cO_2$)  180
56  Oxygen Content: Mixed Venous ($C_{\bar{v}}O_2$)  182
57  Oxygen Duration of E Cylinder  184
58  Oxygen Duration of H or K Cylinder  187
59  Oxygen Duration of Liquid System  190

60  Oxygen Extraction Ratio ($O_2ER$)  195

61  Partial Pressure of a Dry Gas  198

62  $PCO_2$ to $H_2CO_3$  200

63  pH (Henderson-Hasselbalch)  202

64  Poiseuille's Law  205

65  Predicted $P_aO_2$ Based on Age  207

66  Relative Humidity  209

67  Reynolds' Number  212

68  Shunt Equation ($\dot{Q}_{sp}/\dot{Q}_T$): Classic Physiologic  214

69  Shunt Equation ($\dot{Q}_{sp}/\dot{Q}_T$): Estimated  218

70  Shunt Equation: Modified  222

71  Stroke Volume ($SV$) and Stroke Volume Index ($SVI$)  224

72  Stroke Work: Left Ventricular ($LVSW$) and Index ($LVSWI$)  227

73  Stroke Work: Right Ventricular ($RVSW$) and Index ($RVSWI$)  231

74  Temperature Conversion (°C to °F)  234

75  Temperature Conversion (°C to K)  236

76  Temperature Conversion (°F to °C)  238

77  Tidal Volume Based on Flow and $I$ Time  240

78  Time Constant  242

79  Vascular Resistance: Pulmonary  244

80  Vascular Resistance: Systemic  247

81  Ventilator Rate Needed for a Desired $P_aCO_2$  250

82  Weaning Index: Rapid Shallow Breathing ($RSBWI$)  254

83  Weaning Index: Simplified ($SWI$)  257

**Section 3  Basic Statistics and Educational Calculations  261**

Statistics Terminology  263

Measures of Central Tendency  268

Test Reliability  275

Cut Score: Revised Nedelsky Procedure  279

**Section 4  Answer Key to Self-Assessment Questions  283**

**Section 5  Symbols and Abbreviations  291**

Symbols and Abbreviations Commonly Used in Respiratory Physiology  293

**Section 6  Units of Measurement  297**

Pressure Conversions  299

French (Fr) and Millimeter (mm) Conversions  299

Conversions of Conventional and Système International (SI) Units  300

Conversions of Other Units of Measurement  301

**Appendices  305**

A  Partial Pressure (in mm Hg) of Gases in the Air, Alveoli, and Blood  307

B  $P_AO_2$ at Selected $F_IO_2$  307

C  Normal Electrolyte Concentrations in Plasma  308

D  Oxygen Transport Normal Ranges  308

E  Factors for Converting Gas Volumes from ATPS to BTPS  309

F  DuBois Body Surface Chart  310

G  Hemodynamic Normal Ranges  311

H  Periodic Chart of Elements  313

I  Humidity Capacity of Saturated Gas at Selected Temperatures  314

J  Normal Values for Lung Volumes, Capacities, and Ventilation  315

K  Conversion Factors for Calculating Duration of Gas Cylinders  315

L  Barometric Pressures at Selected Altitudes  316

M  Using the Logarithm Table  316

**Bibliography  321**

**Index by Alphabetical Listing  323**

# Listing by Subject Areas

## ACID-BASE

4   Anion Gap   16

8   Bicarbonate Corrections of Base Deficit   25

62   $PCO_2$ to $H_2CO_3$   200

63   pH (Henderson-Hasselbalch)   202

Appendix C: Normal Electrolyte Concentrations in Plasma

## DRUG DOSAGE

20   Dosage Calculation: Intravenous Solution Infusion Dosage   57

21   Dosage Calculation: Intravenous Solution Infusion Rate   60

22   Dosage Calculation: Percent (%) Solutions   63

23   Dosage Calculation: Unit Dose   67

24   Dosage Estimation for Children: Young's Rule   72

25   Dosage Estimation for Infants and Children: Clark's Rule   74

26   Dosage Estimation for Infants and Children: Fried's Rule   76

## GAS THERAPY

2   Alveolar-Arterial Oxygen Tension Gradient $P(A-a)O_2$   11

3   Alveolar Oxygen Tension ($P_AO_2$)   14

5   Arterial/Alveolar Oxygen Tension ($a/A$) Ratio   18

7   ATPS to BTPS   23

16   Correction Factor   45

17   Dalton's Law of Partial Pressure   49

19   Density ($D$) of Gases   54

29   Fick's Law of Diffusion   83

30   $F_IO_2$ from Two Gas Sources   86

31   $F_IO_2$ Needed for a Desired $P_aO_2$   89

32   $F_IO_2$ Needed for a Desired $P_aO_2$ (COPD Patients)   91

37   Gas Law Equations   120

38   Gas Volume Corrections   123

39   Graham's Law of Diffusion Coefficient   126

40   Helium/Oxygen (He/$O_2$) Flow Rate Conversion   128

41   Humidity Deficit   130

52   Oxygen:Air ($O_2$:Air) Entrainment Ratio   168

57   Oxygen Duration of E Cylinder   184

58   Oxygen Duration of H or K Cylinder   187

59   Oxygen Duration of Liquid System   190

61   Partial Pressure of a Dry Gas   198

64   Poiseuille's Law   205

65   Predicted $P_aO_2$ Based on Age   207

67   Reynolds' Number   212

Appendix A: Partial Pressure (in mm Hg) of Gases in the Air, Alveoli, and Blood   307

Appendix B: $P_AO_2$ at Selected $F_IO_2$   307

Appendix E: Factors for Converting Gas Volumes from ATPS to BTPS   309

Appendix I: Humidity Capacity of Saturated Gas at Selected Temperatures   314

Appendix K: Conversion Factors for Calculating Duration of Gas Cylinders   315

## HEMODYNAMIC

9   Body Surface Area   27

10   Cardiac Index (CI)   29

11   Cardiac Output (CO) Fick's Estimated Method   32

46   Mean Arterial Pressure ($MAP$)   151

53   Oxygen Consumption ($\dot{V}O_2$) and Index ($\dot{V}O_2$ Index)   172

60   Oxygen Extraction Ratio ($O_2$ER)   195

68   Shunt Equation ($Q_{sp}/\dot{Q}_T$): Classic Physiologic   214

69   Shunt Equation ($Q_{sp}/\dot{Q}_T$): Estimated   218

70   Shunt Equation: Modified   222

71   Stroke Volume ($SV$) and Stroke Volume Index ($SVI$)   224

72   Stroke Work: Left Ventricular ($LVSW$) and Index ($LVSWI$)   227

73   Stroke Work: Right Ventricular ($RVSW$) and Index ($RVSWI$)   231

79   Vascular Resistance: Pulmonary   244

80   Vascular Resistance: Systemic   247

Appendix G: Hemodynamic Normal Ranges   311

## OXYGEN CONTENT

6   Arterial–Mixed Venous Oxygen Content Difference $[C(a-\bar{v})O_2]$   20

54   Oxygen Content: Arterial ($C_aO_2$)   176

55   Oxygen Content: End-Capillary ($C_cO_2$)   180

56   Oxygen Content: Mixed Venous ($C\bar{v}C_2$)   182

Appendix D: Oxygen Transport Normal Ranges   308

**REFERENCE**

Section 3   Basic Statistics and Educational Calculations   261

  Statistics Terminology   263

  Measures of Central Tendency   268

  Test Reliability   275

  Cut Score: Revised Nedelsky Procedure   279

Section 5: Symbols and Abbreviations   291

Section 6: Units of Measurement   297

Appendix F: DuBois Body Surface Chart   310

Appendix H: Periodic Chart of Elements   313

Appendix L: Barometric Pressures at Selected Altitudes   316

Appendix M: Using the Logarithm Table and Common Logarithms of Numbers   317

Bibliography   321

Index by Alphabetical Listing   323

**REVIEW**

Section 1: Review of Basic Math Functions   1

Section 4: Answer Key to Self-Assessment Questions   283

**TEMPERATURE CONVERSIONS**

74   Temperature Conversion (°C to °F)   234

75   Temperature Conversion (°C to K)   236

76   Temperature Conversion (°F to °C)   238

**VENTILATION**

1   Airway Resistance: Estimated ($R_{aw}$)   9

12   Compliance: Dynamic ($C_{dyn}$)   35

13   Compliance: Static ($C_{st}$)   38

14   Compliance: Total ($C_T$)   41

15   Corrected Tidal Volume ($V_T$)   43

18   Deadspace to Tidal Volume Ratio ($V_D/V_T$)   51

27   Elastance ($E$)   78

28   Endotracheal Tube Size for Children   80

33   Flow Rate in Mechanical Ventilation   93

42   $I{:}E$ Ratio   132

43   Law of LaPlace   138

44   Lung Volumes and Capacities   140

45   Mean Airway Pressure ($MAWP$)   147

50   Minute Ventilation during IMV   162

51   Minute Ventilation: Expired and Alveolar   164

77   Tidal Volume Based on Flow and $I$ Time   240

78   Time Constant   242

81   Ventilator Rate Needed for a Desired $P_aCO_2$   250

82   Weaning Index: Rapid Shallow Breathing ($RSBWI$)   254

83   Weaning Index: Simplified ($SWI$)   257

Appendix J: Normal Values for Lung Volumes, Capacities, and Ventilation   315

# Preface

A tool can only be as useful as the way it is used. There is much truth to this statement in respiratory care calculations. Respiratory care equations are some of the most useful tools we use, directly or indirectly, in clinical practice. When an equation is properly applied to the clinical setting and correctly calculated, the answer can be interpreted in a meaningful way. Our patients benefit from it.

Each and every mathematical equation integrates many variables into a broad but interrelated idea. In a classroom setting, equations allow the student to learn the appropriate applications of concepts in respiratory care. In a clinical setting, equations can be used as an adjunct to the application of respiratory care equipment and procedures.

Modern respiratory care equipment and testing protocols are designed to provide instantaneous answers, charts, and graphs. But an understanding of how these outputs come about is nevertheless a prerequisite to proper interpretation of the data provided by the tools we use in patient care.

The purpose of this book is to provide a clear and concise reference source for respiratory care calculations. It is intended for use in classroom, laboratory, and clinical settings by respiratory care practitioners and other health care providers. Each equation presented in this workbook is accompanied by a description of the abbreviations. It is followed by an example of its calculation. Any pertinent clinical notes are then described. At the end of each topic, practice exercises are included to reinforce learning and retention.

The section on review of basic mathematical functions should be useful for a quick review of calculations and the interrelationship of variables in an equation. As the self-assessment questions follow the examination format of the National Board for Respiratory Care (NBRC) certification and written registry examinations, they are useful in preparing for the national board examinations. While all the respiratory care equations presented can be used as stand-alone units, Sections 3, 5, and 6 and the appendices at the end of this book are a useful reference source for many other respiratory care applications.

David W. Chang

# Acknowledgments

I want to express my appreciation to the following educators and colleagues for their careful review of the revised manuscript. They pointed out areas in the first edition that needed clarification and provided useful comments for this new edition. Their suggestions made this book more organized as a student workbook and more complete as a reference source for clinical practice. The reviewers are:

Sharon A. Baer, MBA, RRT, CPFT
Program Director, Respiratory Care
Naugatuck Valley College
Waterbury, Connecticut

Leanna Konechne, MEd, RRT
Program Director, Respiratory Care
Pima Medical Institute
Tucson, Arizona

Diana L. Luder, DPA, RRT
Program Director
Respiratory Care Practitioner Program
Northeast Wisconsin Technical College
Green Bay, Wisconsin

Candace S. Schladenhauffen, BS, RRT, RPFT, RCP
Program Chair, Respiratory Care
Ivy Tech State College
Fort Wayne, Indiana

For their scrupulous attention to all details and corrections in this new edition, I extend my gratitude to Dawn Gerrain, Acquisitions Editor, Debra Flis, Development Editor, John Mickelbank, Production Coordinator, and Vin Berger, Art Coordinator, of Delmar Publishers and to Otto Barz, Deborah Constantine, and George Ernsberger of Publishing Synthesis Ltd., New York.

Dr. Donald F. Egan's contributions to and knowledge in the field of respiratory care are legendary. I am especially grateful for his comments and the Foreword written for the first edition of this book. I wish him well and a tranquil retirement in North Carolina.

David W. Chang

*Dedicated to*
*my mother, Tsung-yuin,*
*and to my uncle Jim, and my wife, Bonnie*

# 1

# Review of

# Basic Math

# Functions

# Review of
# Basic Math Functions

**1.** Add numbers with decimal.

*Note:* Line up the decimals properly.

**EXAMPLE**     $43.45 + 10.311 + 0.25 = 54.011$

$$\begin{array}{r} 43.45 \\ 10.311 \\ +\ \ 0.25 \\ \hline 54.011 \end{array}$$

**2.** Subtract numbers with decimal.

*Note:* Line up the decimals properly.

**EXAMPLE**     $198.24 - 40.015 = 158.225$

$$\begin{array}{r} 198.24 \\ -\ \ 40.015 \\ \hline 158.225 \end{array}$$

**3.** Multiply numbers with decimal.

*Note:* Count the total number of digits after the decimals in the numbers and place the decimal in the answer accordingly.

**EXAMPLE**     $50.6 \times 0.002 = 0.1012$ can be treated as

$$\begin{array}{r} 506 \\ \times\ \ \ 2 \\ \hline 1{,}012 \end{array}$$

There are a total of 4 digits (1 in 50.6 + 3 in 0.002) after the decimals in the numbers. The decimal in the product 1,012 comes after the 2 ($1{,}012 = 1{,}012.0$); moving it 4 places to the left gives an answer of 0.1012.

**4.** Divide numbers with decimal.

*Terminology:* $\dfrac{\text{Dividend}}{\text{Divisor}} = \text{Answer}$

*Step 1.* Count and compare the number of digits after the decimal in the dividend and that after the decimal in the divisor.

*Step 2.* Move the decimal points for both dividend and divisor to the right so that they become whole numbers. Remember to move decimals the same number of places to the right.

## EXAMPLE

$\dfrac{0.68}{3.4}$ can be changed to $\dfrac{68}{340} = 0.2$

Move the decimal points two places to the right for both the dividend and the divisor. (0.68 is changed to 68 and 3.4 is changed to 340.)

## EXAMPLE

$\dfrac{2.4}{0.006}$ can be changed to $\dfrac{2400}{6} = 400$

Move the decimal points three places to the right for the dividend and the divisor. (2.4 is changed to 2400 and 0.006 is changed to 6.)

**5.**  Add / subtract and multiply / divide

*Note:* Perform multiplication / division **before** addition / subtraction.

## EXAMPLE 1

$$12 \times 6 - 2 = (12 \times 6) - 2$$
$$= 72 - 2$$
$$= 70$$

## EXAMPLE 2

$$116 - \dfrac{445}{5} = 116 - \left(\dfrac{455}{5}\right)$$
$$= 116 - 91$$
$$= 25$$

**6.**  Parentheses

*Note:* Perform calculation within parentheses in the order ( ), [ ], and { }.

## EXAMPLE 1

$$12 \times (6 - 2) = 12 \times 4$$
$$= 48$$

## EXAMPLE 2

$$194 - \{ [20 \times (9 - 5)] + 14 \} = 194 - \{[20 \times 4] + 14\}$$
$$= 194 - \{80 + 14\}$$
$$= 194 - 94$$
$$= 100$$

**7.**  Ratio

*Note:* A ratio compares two related quantities, or measurements. It is usually expressed in the form 1:2, as in *I:E* ratio.

## EXAMPLE 1

*I:E* ratio of 1:2 means that the expiratory phase (*E*) is two times as long as the inspiratory phase (*I*). A ratio is dimensionless: it does not provide units such as seconds or inches. An *I:E* ratio of 1:2 may mean that the inspiratory time (*I* time) is 1 second and expiratory time (*E* time) is 2 seconds *or* the *I* time is 2 seconds and the *E* time is 4 seconds.

**EXAMPLE 2**    Inverse *I:E* ratio of 2:1 means that the inspiratory phase is two times as long as the expiratory phase.

**EXAMPLE 3**    Oxygen:air entrainment ratio of 1:4 means that 1 part of oxygen is combined with 4 parts of air.

**8.**    Percentage

*Note:* Percentage expresses a value in parts of 100. It is written in the form 65% or 0.65, as in $F_IO_2$.

**EXAMPLE 1**    An intrapulmonary shunt of 15% means that 15 of 100 units of perfusion do not take part in gas exchange.

**EXAMPLE 2**    An arterial oxygen content of 21 vol% means that 21 of 100 units of arterial blood are saturated with oxygen.

**9.**    Relationships of *X* and *Y* in equation $A = \dfrac{X}{Y}$ *

[When *A* is constant, *X* and *Y* are directly related]

**EXAMPLE 1**    $$\text{Resistance} = \frac{\text{Pressure change } (\Delta P)}{\text{Flow}}$$

When airway resistance is constant, an **increase** in driving pressure generates a **higher** flow. Likewise, a **decrease** in driving pressure yields a **lower** flow.

**EXAMPLE 2**    $$\text{Compliance} = \frac{\text{Volume change } (\Delta V)}{\text{Pressure change } (\Delta P)}$$

When compliance is constant, an **increase** in pressure generates a **higher** lung volume. By the same token, a **decrease** in pressure **lowers** the lung volume.

---

*$A = \dfrac{X}{Y}$ can be rewritten as $X = AY$ or $Y = \dfrac{X}{A}$. When any two of three values are known, the third can be calculated.

**10.** Relationships of $A$ and $X$ in equation $A = \dfrac{X}{Y}$

[When $Y$ is constant, $A$ and $X$ are directly related]

## EXAMPLE 1

$$\text{Resistance} = \frac{\text{Pressure change } (\Delta P)}{\text{Flow}}$$

In order to maintain a constant flow, an **increase** in driving pressure is needed to overcome a **higher** resistance. If the resistance is **low**, **less** pressure is needed to maintain a constant flow.

## EXAMPLE 2

$$\text{Compliance} = \frac{\text{Volume change } (\Delta V)}{\text{Pressure change } (\Delta P)}$$

When a constant peak inspiratory pressure is used on a pressure-limited ventilator (e.g., IPPB), the volume delivered is **increased** in the presence of **high** compliance. On the other hand, the volume delivered by a pressure-limited ventilator is **decreased** with **low** compliance.

**11.** Relationships of $A$ and $Y$ in equation $A = \dfrac{X}{Y}$

[When $X$ is constant, $A$ and $Y$ are inversely related]

## EXAMPLE 1

$$\text{Resistance} = \frac{\text{Pressure change } (\Delta P)}{\text{Flow}}$$

In the presence of **increasing** airway resistance, air flow to the lungs is **decreased** if the pressure (work of breathing or ventilator work) remains constant. On the other hand, with **decreasing** airway resistance, air flow to the lungs is **increased** at constant pressure (work of breathing or ventilator work).

## EXAMPLE 2

$$\text{Compliance} = \frac{\text{Volume change } (\Delta V)}{\text{Pressure change } (\Delta P)}$$

When a constant tidal volume is used on a volume-limited ventilator, the peak inspiratory pressure of the ventilator **increases** in the presence of **decreasing** compliance. As the compliance **improves** (**increases**), the inspiratory pressure **decreases**.

**12.** Relationships of $A, B$ and $X, Y$ in equation $\dfrac{A}{B} = \dfrac{X}{Y}$ [same as $AY = BX$]

[$A$ or $Y$ is directly related to $B$ or $X$. $A$ and $Y$ are inversely related to each other]

[$B$ or $X$ is directly related to $A$ or $Y$. $B$ and $X$ are inversely related to each other]

# 2

# Respiratory Care

# Calculations

CHAPTER

# 1

# Airway Resistance: Estimated ($R_{aw}$)

## EQUATION

$$R_{aw} = \frac{(P_{max} - P_{st})}{Flow} \text{ *}$$

| | | |
|---|---|---|
| $R_{aw}$ | : | Airway resistance in cm $H_2O$ / L / sec. |
| $P_{max}$ | : | Maximum airway pressure in cm $H_2O$ (peak airway pressure). |
| $P_{st}$ | : | Static airway pressure in cm $H_2O$ (plateau airway pressure). |
| Flow | : | Flow rate in L / sec. |

## NORMAL VALUE

0.6 to 2.4 cm $H_2O$ / L / sec at flow rate of 0.5 L / sec (30 L / min). If the patient is intubated, use serial measurements to establish trend.

## EXAMPLE

Calculate the estimated airway resistance of a patient whose peak airway pressure is 25 cm $H_2O$ and whose plateau pressure is 10 cm $H_2O$. The ventilator flow rate is set at 60 L / min (1 L / sec).

$$R_{aw} = \frac{(P_{max} - P_{st})}{Flow}$$

$$= \frac{(25 - 10)}{1}$$

$$= \frac{15}{1}$$

$$= 15 \text{ cm } H_2O / L / sec$$

## EXERCISE

Given: Peak airway pressure = 45 cm $H_2O$
Plateau pressure = 35 cm $H_2O$
Inspiratory flow = 50 L / min (0.83 L / sec)
Calculate the estimated airway resistance.

### NOTES

This equation estimates the airway resistance of an intubated patient on a volume ventilator. ($P_{max} - P_{st}$) represents the pressure gradient in the presence of flow.

In ventilators with square-wave flow patterns, the inspiratory flow rate can be used in this equation. Otherwise, a pneumotachometer may be needed to measure the inspiratory flow rate during $P_{max}$. Flow rates in L/min should first be changed to L/sec by dividing L/min by 60. For example:

$$40 \text{ L/min} = \frac{40 \text{ (L/min)}}{60}$$
$$= 0.67 \text{ L/sec}$$

Some conditions leading to an increase in airway resistance include bronchospasm, retained secretions, and use of a small endotracheal or tracheostomy tube. These increases in airway resistance can be minimized by using bronchodilators for bronchospasm, frequent suctioning for retained secretions, and the largest appropriate endotracheal or tracheostomy tube.

[Answer: $R_{aw}$ = 12 cm $H_2O$/L/sec]

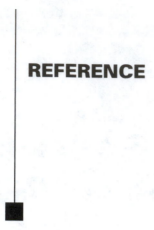

**REFERENCE**

Burton

*In nonintubated subjects, a body plethysmography must be used to measure and calculate the airway resistance by:* $R_{aw} = \dfrac{(P_{ao} - P_{alv})}{Flow}$, *where $P_{ao}$ is the pressure at the airway opening and $P_{alv}$ is the pressure in the alveoli.*

## SELF-ASSESSMENT QUESTIONS

1a.   Calculate the estimated airway resistance ($R_{aw_{est}}$) of a patient whose peak airway pressure is 60 cm $H_2O$ and plateau pressure is 40 cm $H_2O$. The ventilator flow rate is set at 60 L/min (1 L/sec).
(A) 10 cm $H_2O$/L/sec
(B) 20 cm $H_2O$/L/sec
(C) 40 cm $H_2O$/L/sec
(D) 50 cm $H_2O$/L/sec
(E) 60 cm $H_2O$/L/sec

1b.   When a volume-limited ventilator is used, the peak airway pressure is directly related to the
(A) patient's airway resistance.
(B) patient's lung compliance.
(C) respiratory rate.
(D) $F_IO_2$.
(E) oxygen saturation reading.

# CHAPTER

# 2

# Alveolar–Arterial Oxygen Tension Gradient: $P(A-a)O_2$

## EQUATION

$P(A-a)O_2 = P_AO_2 - P_aO_2$

$P(A-a)O_2$ : Alveolar-arterial oxygen tension gradient in mm Hg.
$P_AO_2$ : Alveolar-arterial oxygen tension in mm Hg.*
$P_aO_2$ : Arterial oxygen tension in mm Hg.

### NOTE

The value of $P(A-a)O_2$ (also known as $A-a$ gradient) can be used to estimate (1) the degree of hypoxemia and (2) the degree of physiologic shunt. It is derived from a less commonly used shunt equation:

$$\frac{Q_s}{Q_T} = \frac{(P_AO_2 - P_aO_2) \times 0.003}{(C_aO_2 - C_{\bar{v}}O_2) + (P_AO_2 - P_aO_2) \times 0.003}$$

The $P(A-a)O_2$ is increased when hypoxemia is due to $\frac{V}{Q}$ mismatch, diffusion defect, or shunt. In the absence of cardiopulmonary disease, it increases with aging.

## NORMAL VALUE

(1) On *room* air, the $P(A-a)O_2$ should be less than 4 mm Hg for every 10 years in age. For example, the $P(A-a)O_2$ should be less than 24 mm Hg for a 60-year-old patient.
(2) On *100% oxygen*, every 50 mm Hg difference in $P(A-a)O_2$ approximates 2% shunt.

## EXAMPLE 1

Given: $P_AO_2$   = 100 mm Hg
        $P_aO_2$   = 85 mm Hg
        $F_IO_2$   = 21%
        Patient age = 40 years
Calculate $P(A-a)O_2$. Is it or abnormal for this patient?

$P(A-a)O_2$  = $P_AO_2 - P_aO_2$
          = $(100-85)$ mm Hg
          = 15 mm Hg

$P(A-a)O_2$ of 15 mm Hg is normal for a 40-year-old patient.

## EXAMPLE 2

Given: $P_AO_2$ = 660 mm Hg
        $P_aO_2$ = 360 mm Hg
        $F_IO_2$ = 100%
Calculate $P(A-a)O_2$. What is the estimated physiologic shunt in percent?

$P(A-a)O_2$ = $P_AO_2 - P_aO_2$
          = $(660-360)$ mm Hg
          = 300 mm Hg

Since every 50 mm Hg difference in $P(A-a)O_2$ approximates 2% shunt, 300 mm Hg $P(A-a)O_2$ difference is estimated to be 12% shunt:

$$\frac{300}{50} \times 2 = 6 \times 12 = 12.$$

## EXERCISE 1

Given: $P_AO_2$ = 93 mm Hg
$P_aO_2$ = 60 mm Hg
$F_IO_2$ = 21%
Patient age = 65 years
Calculate $P(A-a)O_2$.
Is the $P(A-a)O_2$ normal or abnormal for this patient?

[Answer: $P(A-a)O_2$ = 33 mm Hg. It is abnormal since 33 mm Hg is more than 26 mm Hg, the allowable difference for patient's age.]

## EXERCISE 2

Given: $P_AO_2$ = 646 mm Hg
$P_aO_2$ = 397 mm Hg
$F_IO_2$ = 100%
Calculate the $P(A-a)O_2$ and estimate the percent physiologic shunt.

[Answer: $P(A-a)O_2$ = 249 mm Hg. The estimated shunt is 10% since every 50 mm Hg $P(A-a)O_2$ difference represents about 2% shunt:

$$\frac{249}{50} \times 2 = 5 \times 2 = 10.$$

## REFERENCES

Barnes; Burton; Shapiro (1)

## SEE

*Arterial/Alveolar Oxygen Tension (a/A) Ratio.*

*\*See Alveolar Oxygen Tension ($P_AO_2$) for calculation of $P_AO_2$.*

# SELF-ASSESSMENT QUESTIONS

2a.  Given the following values for room air: $P_AO_2 = 105$ mm Hg, $P_aO_2 = 70$ mm Hg. What is the $P(A-a)O_2$? Is it normal for a 70-year-old patient?

(A) 70 mm Hg; normal

(B) 70 mm Hg; abnormal

(C) 35 mm Hg; normal

(D) 35 mm Hg; abnormal

(E) 105 mm Hg; normal

2b.  If a patient's $P_aO_2$ is 70 mm Hg and $P(A-a)O_2$ is 30 mm Hg, what is the $P_AO_2$?

(A) 30 mm Hg

(B) 40 mm Hg

(C) 70 mm Hg

(D) 100 mm Hg

(E) 159 mm Hg

2c.  Given: $P_AO_2 = 638$ mm Hg; $P_aO_2 = 240$ mm Hg, $F_IO_2 = 100\%$. What is the calculated $P(A-a)O_2$ and the estimated physiologic shunt?

(A) 240 mm Hg; 12%

(B) 240 mm Hg; 16%

(C) 398 mm Hg; 16%

(D) 398 mm Hg; 22%

(E) 638 mm Hg; 22%

2d.  A patient has a $P_aO_2$ of 540 mm Hg on 100% oxygen. If the $P_AO_2$ is 642 mm Hg, what is the alveolar-arterial oxygen tension difference? What is the estimated shunt based on this difference?

(A) 102 mm Hg; 2%

(B) 102 mm Hg; 4%

(C) 540 mm Hg; 4%

(D) 540 mm Hg; 8%

(E) 642 mm Hg; 84%

# CHAPTER

# 3

# Alveolar Oxygen Tension ($P_AO_2$)

## NOTE

$P_AO_2$ is primarily used for other calculations such as alveolar–arterial oxygen tension gradient ($A-a$ gradient) and arterial/alveolar oxygen tension ($a$/A) ratio. The $P_AO_2$ value is directly proportional to the $F_IO_2$. Under normal conditions, a higher $F_IO_2$ gives a higher $P_AO_2$ value and vice versa.

## EQUATION

$$P_AO_2 = (P_B - PH_2O) \times F_IO_2 - P_aCO_2 \times 1.25)^*$$

$P_AO_2$ : Alveolar oxygen tension in mm Hg.

$P_B$ : Barometric pressure in mm Hg.

$PH_2O$ : Water vapor pressure, 47 mm Hg saturated at 37 °C

$F_IO_2$ : Inspired oxygen concentration in percent.

$P_aCO_2$ : Arterial carbon dioxide tension in mm Hg.

1.25 : $\dfrac{1}{0.8} \left( \dfrac{1}{\text{Normal respiratory exchange ratio}} \right)$ ;

*this ratio is omitted when $F_IO_2$ is greater than 60%.

## NORMAL VALUE

The normal values vary according to the $F_IO_2$.

## EXAMPLE

Given: $P_B$ = 760 mm Hg

$PH_2O$ = 47 mm Hg

$F_IO_2$ = 40% or 0.4

$P_aCO_2$ = 30 mm Hg

$P_AO_2$ = $(P_B - PH_2O) \times F_IO_2 - (P_aCO_2 \times 1.25)$

= $(760 - 47) \times 0.4 - (30 \times 1.25)$

= $713 \times 0.4 - 37.5$

= $285.2 - 37.5$

= 247.7 or 248 mm Hg

## EXERCISE

Given: $P_B$ = 750 mm Hg

$PH_2O$ = 47 mm Hg

$F_IO_2$ = 50% or 0.5

$P_aCO_2$ = 40 mm Hg

Calculate the $P_AO_2$.

[Answer: $P_AO_2$ = 301.5 or 302 mm Hg]

**REFERENCES**  Madama; Ruppel; Shapiro (1)

**SEE**  *Appendix A, partial Pressure (in mm Hg) of Gases in the Air, Alveoli, and Blood; and Appendix B, $P_AO_2$ at Selected $F_IO_2$.*

*Modified from: $P_AO_2 = (P_B - PH_2O) \times F_IO_2 - P_aCO_2 \times [F_IO_2 + \dfrac{(1 - F_IO_2)}{R}]$, where R is the respiratory exchange ratio, normally 0.8.*

## SELF-ASSESSMENT QUESTIONS

3a.  Which of the following is the clinical equation to calculate the partial pressure of oxygen in the alveoli?

(A) $P_AO_2 = (P_B - PH_2O) \times F_IO_2 - (P_aCO_2 \times 1.25)$

(B) $P_AO_2 = (P_B - PH_2O) \times F_IO_2$

(C) $P_AO_2 = (P_B \times F_IO_2) - (P_aCO_2 - PH_2O)$

(D) $P_AO_2 = (P_B \times F_IO_2) - PH_2O$

(E) $P_AO_2 = P_B - PH_2O - P_aCO_2 - PN_2$

3b.  Given: $P_B = 760$ mm Hg, $PH_2O = 47$ mm Hg, $F_IO_2 = 0.7$, $P_aCO_2 = 50$ mm Hg. The $P_AO_2$ is about [Do not use respiratory exchange ratio in equation since $F_IO_2$ is greater than 60%].

(A) 403 mm Hg.

(B) 417 mm Hg.

(C) 428 mm Hg.

(D) 449 mm Hg.

(E) 451 mm Hg.

3c.  Calculate the alveolar oxygen tension ($P_AO_2$) given the following values: $P_B = 750$ mm Hg, $PH_2O = 47$ mm Hg, $F_IO_2 = 30\%$ or 0.3, and $P_aCO_2 = 40$ mm Hg.

(A) 30 mm Hg

(B) 100 mm Hg

(C) 161 mm Hg

(D) 170 mm Hg

(E) 185 mm Hg

3d.  Given: $P_B = 760$ mm Hg, $PH_2O = 47$ mm Hg, $F_IO_2 = 70\%$ or 0.7, and $P_aCO_2 = 40$ mm Hg. What is the calculated alveolar oxygen tension ($P_AO_2$)? [Do not use respiratory exchange ratio in equation since $F_IO_2$ is greater than 60%]

(A) 70 mm Hg

(B) 100 mm Hg

(C) 449 mm Hg

(D) 459 mm Hg

(E) 713 mm Hg

# CHAPTER

# 4
# Anion Gap

Anion gap helps to evaluate the overall electrolyte balance between the cations and anions in the extracellular fluid. Potassium is not included in the calculation because it contributes little to the extracellular cation concentration. If potassium is included in the equation, the normal value range would be 15 to 20 mEq/L.

Metabolic acidosis in the presence of a *normal anion gap* is usually caused by a loss of base. It is known as hyperchloremia metabolic acidosis because this condition is usually related to excessive accumulation of chloride ions.

Metabolic acidosis in the presence of an *increased anion gap* is usually due to increased fixed acids. These fixed acids may be produced (e.g., renal failure, diabetic ketoacidosis, lactic acidosis), or they may be added to the body (e.g., poisoning by salicylates and alcohols).

Fluid and electrolyte therapy is indicated when there is a significant anion gap ( > 16 mEq/L).

## EQUATION

$$\text{Anion gap} = Na^+ - (Cl^- + HCO_3^-)$$

$Na^+$ : Serum sodium concentration in mEq/L.

$Cl^-$ : Serum chloride concentration in mEq/L.

$HCO_3^-$: Serum bicarbonate concentration in mEq/L.*

## NORMAL VALUE

10 to 14 mEq/L

15 to 20 mEq/L if potassium ($K^+$) is included in the equation

## EXAMPLE

Given: $Na^+$ = 140 mEq/L

$Cl^-$ = 105 mEq/L

$HCO_3^-$ = 22 mEq/L

Calculate the anion gap.

$$
\begin{aligned}
\text{Anion gap} &= Na^+ - (Cl^- + HCO_3^-) \\
&= 140 - (105 + 22) \\
&= 140 - 127 \\
&= 13 \text{ mEq/L}
\end{aligned}
$$

## EXERCISE

Given: $Na^+$ = 130 mEq/L

$Cl^-$ = 92 mEq/L

$HCO_3^-$ = 20 mEq/L

What is the calculated anion gap?

[Answer: Anion gap = 18 mEq/L]

## REFERENCES

Kacmarek; Malasanos; Malley; Wilkins

## SEE

*Appendix C, Normal Electrolyte Concentrations in Plasma.*

*Total $CO_2$ is sometimes used in place of $HCO_3^-$. Normal range is 11 to 15 mEq/L if total $CO_2$ is used.*

## SELF-ASSESSMENT QUESTIONS

4a. A physician asks you to evaluate a patient's overall status of electrolyte balance. You would use the following set of electrolyes to calculate the anion gap:

(A) $Na^+, H^+, Cl^-, HCO_3^-$

(B) $Na^+, K^+, HCO_3^-$

(C) $Na^+, Cl^-, HCO_3^-$

(D) $Na^+, Ca^{++}, Cl^-, HCO_3^-$

(E) $Na^+, Cl^-, HCO_3^-, SO_4^-$

4b. Given: $Na^+ = 138$ mEq/L, $Cl^- = 102$ mEq/L, $HCO_3^- = 25$ mEq/L. Calculate the anion gap.

(A) 36 mEq/L

(B) 25 mEq/L

(C) 12 mEq/L

(D) 11 mEq/L

(E) 0 mEq/L

4c. Given: $Na^+ = 135$ mEq/L, $Cl^- = 96$ mEq/L, $HCO_3^- = 22$ mEq/L. What is the calculated anion gap?

(A) 15 mEq/L

(B) 17 mEq/L

(C) 20 mEq/L

(D) 22 mEq/L

(E) 30 mEq/L

# 5

# Arterial/Alveolar Oxygen Tension (*a/A*) Ratio

*NOTE*

The *a/A* ratio is an indicator of the efficiency of oxygen transport. A low *a/A* ratio reflects ventilation/perfusion (*V/Q*) mismatch, diffusion defect, or shunt.

This ratio is often used to calculate the approximate $F_IO_2$ needed to obtain a desired $P_aO_2$.

## EQUATION

$$a/A \text{ ratio} = \frac{P_aO_2}{P_AO_2}$$

$a/A$ ratio : Arterial/alveolar oxygen tension ratio in percent.

$P_aO_2$ : Arterial oxygen tension in mm Hg.

$P_AO_2$ : Alveolar oxygen tension in mm Hg.*

## NORMAL VALUE

>60%

## EXAMPLE

Calculate the $a/A$ ratio if the $P_aO_2 = 100$ mm Hg and $P_AO_2 = 248$ mm Hg.

$$a/A \text{ ratio} = \frac{P_aO_2}{P_AO_2}$$

$$= \frac{100}{248}$$

$$= 0.403 \text{ or } 40\%$$

## EXERCISE

Given: $P_AO_2 = 320$ mm Hg

$P_aO_2 = 112$ mm Hg

Calculate the $a/A$ ratio.

[Answer: $a/A$ ratio = 0.35 or 35%]

## REFERENCES

Burton; Krider

## SEE

*Alveolar–Arterial Oxygen Tension Gradient: $P(A-a)O_2$; $F_IO_2$ Needed for a Desired $P_aO_2$.*

*Refer to Alveolar Oxygen Tension ($P_AO_2$) for calculation of $P_AO_2$.*

## SELF-ASSESSMENT QUESTIONS

5a.    Calculate the $a/A$ ratio if the $P_aO_2 = 80$ mm Hg and $P_AO_2 = 170$ mm Hg.

(A)  47%

(B)  80%

(C)  212%

(D)  90 mm Hg

(E)  250 mm Hg

5b.    Given: $P_AO_2 = 210$ mm Hg, $P_aO_2 = 45$ mm Hg. Calculate the $a/A$ ratio.

(A)  12%

(B)  21%

(C)  30%

(D)  47%

(E)  76%

# CHAPTER

# 6

# Arterial–Mixed Venous Oxygen Content Difference [C(a – $\bar{v}$)O$_2$]

## *NOTES*

Measurements of arterial–mixed venous oxygen content difference [$C(a-\bar{v})O_2$] are useful in assessing changes in oxygen consumption and cardiac output. Under conditions of normal oxygen consumption and cardiac output, about 25% of the available oxygen is used for tissue metabolism. Therefore, a $C(a-\bar{v})O_2$ of 5 vol% ($C_aO_2$ 20 vol% – $C_{\bar{v}}O_2$ 15 vol%) reflects a balanced relationship between oxygen consumption and cardiac output (Figure 1).

According to the cardiac output equation (Fick's estimated method)

$$\dot{Q}_T = \frac{\dot{V}O_2}{[C(a-\bar{v})O_2]}$$

the arterial–mixed venous oxygen content difference [$C(a-\bar{v})O_2$] is directly related to the oxygen consumption ($\dot{V}O_2$) and inversely related to the cardiac output ($\dot{Q}_T$).

### Relationship of *C*(a – $\bar{v}$)O$_2$ and oxygen consumption

If the *cardiac output* stays unchanged or is unable to compensate for hypoxia, an increase of oxygen consumption (metabolic rate) will cause an increase in $C(a-\bar{v})O_2$. A decrease of oxygen consumption will cause a decrease in $C(a-\bar{v})O_2$.

## EQUATION

$C(a-\bar{v})O_2 = C_aO_2 - C_{\bar{v}}O_2$

$C(a-\bar{v})O_2$:  Arterial–mixed venous oxygen content difference in vol%.

$C_aO_2$  :  Arterial oxygen content in vol%.

$C_{\bar{v}}O_2$  :  Mixed venous oxygen content in vol%.

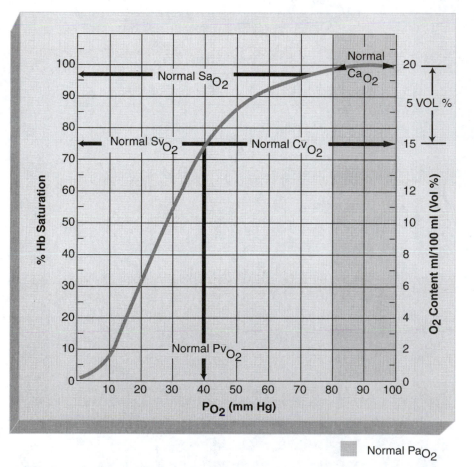

**Figure 1**  *Oxygen dissociation curve. The normal oxygen content difference between arterial and venous blood is about 5 vol%. Note that both the right side and the left side of the graph illustrate that approximately 25 percent of the available oxygen is used for tissue metabolism, and therefore the hemoglobin returning to the lungs is normally about 75 percent saturated with oxygen.*

NOTES *(continued)*

**Relationship of C(a – $\overline{v}$ )O2 and cardiac output**

When *oxygen consumption* remains constant, the $C(a - \overline{v})O_2$ becomes a good indicator of the cardiac output. A decrease of $C(a - \overline{v})O_2$ is indicative of an increase of cardiac output, and an increase of $C(a - \overline{v})O_2$ reflects a decrease of cardiac output.

For a summary of factors that change the $C(a - \overline{v})O_2$ values, see Tables 1 and 2.

**TABLE 1.   Factors That Increase the $C(a - \overline{v})O_2$**

Decreased cardiac output

Periods of increased oxygen consumption

  Exercise

  Seizures

  Shivering in postoperative patient

  Hyperthermia

From Des Jardins, T.R., *Cardiopulmonary Anatomy and Physiology—Essentials for Respiratory Care.* 3rd ed. Albany, NY: Delmar Publishers, 1998.

**TABLE 2.   Factors That Decrease the $C(a - \overline{v})O_2$**

Increased cardiac output

Decreased oxygen consumption

  Skeletal relaxation (e.g., induced by drugs)

  Peripheral shunting (e.g., sepsis, trauma)

  Certain poisons (e.g., cyanide prevents cellular metabolism)

  Hypothermia

Modified from Des Jardins, T.R., *Cardiopulmonary Anatomy and Physiology—Essentials for Respiratory Care.* 3rd ed. Albany, NY: Delmar Publishers, 1998.

## NORMAL VALUES

<5 vol% for healthy or critically ill patients with cardiovascular compensation.

>6 vol% for critically ill patients without cardiovascular compensation.

## EXAMPLE

Given: $C_aO_2 = 18.33$ vol%

$\qquad C_{\overline{v}}O_2 = 14.18$ vol%

$C(a - \overline{v})O_2 = C_aO - C_{\overline{v}}O_2$

$\qquad\qquad = 18.33 - 14.18$

$\qquad\qquad = 4.15$ vol%

## EXERCISE 1

Given: $C_aO_2 = 16.25$ vol%

$\qquad C_{\overline{v}}O_2 = 13.17$ vol%

Calculate the $C(a - \overline{v})O_2$. Is it normal for a critically ill patient?

[Answer: $C(a - \overline{v})O_2 = 3.08$ vol%. Normal for this patient.]

## EXERCISE 2

Given: $C_aO_2 = 16.85$ vol%

$\qquad C_{\overline{v}}O_2 = 10.60$ vol%

Calculate the $C(a - \bar{v})O_2$. Is it normal for a critically ill patient?

[Answer: $C(a - \bar{v})O_2 = 6.25$ vol%. Abnormal for this patient.]

**REFERENCE**  Shapiro (1)

*See also Oxygen Content: Arterial (C$_a$O$_2$); Oxygen Content: Mixed Venous (C$_{\bar{v}}$O$_2$); Appendix D, Oxygen Transport Normal Ranges.*

## SELF-ASSESSMENT QUESTIONS

6a.  The normal arterial–mixed venous oxygen content difference [$C(a - \bar{v})O_2$] is _____ or less.

(A) 20 vol%

(B) 15 vol%

(C) 10 vol%

(D) 5 vol%

(E) 1 vol%

6b.  A critically ill patient has the following oxygen content measurements: $C_aO_2 = 20.5$ vol%, $C_{\bar{v}}O_2 = 16.6$ vol%. What is the arterial–mixed venous oxygen content difference [$C(a - \bar{v})O_2$]? Is it normal for this patient?

(A) 3.9 vol%; normal

(B) 3.9 vol%; abnormal

(C) 37.1 vol%; normal

(D) 37.1 vol%; abnormal

(E) 80.8%; abnormal

6c.  The following oxygen content measurements are obtained from a critically ill patient: $C_cO_2 = 21.0$ vol%, $C_aO_2 = 19.8$ vol%, $C_{\bar{v}}O_2 = 12.8$ vol%. What is the calculated arterial–mixed venous oxygen content difference [$C(a - \bar{v})O_2$? Is it normal for this patient?

(A) 0.2 vol%; normal

(B) 0.2 vol%; abnormal

(C) 7 vol%; normal

(D) 7 vol%; abnormal

(E) insufficient data to calculate value

# CHAPTER

# 7

# ATPS to BTPS

*NOTE*

According to Charles' law, lung volumes and flow rates measured at room temperature should be corrected to reflect the actual values at body temperature. The conversion factors in Appendix E should be used if the pulmonary function device does not correct for the temperature change.

The values shown in Appendix E are accurate for a barometric pressure of 760 mm Hg. At barometric pressures as low as 750 mm Hg, changes in the conversion factors are negligible. If a precise conversion factor is desired at any barometric pressure, use the equation included in Appendix E.

## EQUATION

$Volume_{BTPS} = Volume_{ATPS} \times Factor$

$Volume_{BTPS}$ :  Gas volume saturated with water at body temperature (37 °C) and ambient pressure

$Volume_{ATPS}$ :  Gas volume saturated with water at ambient (room) temperature and pressure

Factor :  Factors for converting gas volumes from ATPS to BTPS (see Appendix E.)

## EXAMPLE

A tidal volume measured under the ATPS condition is 600 mL. What is the corrected volume if the room temperature was 25 °C?

$Volume_{BTPS} = Volume_{ATPS} \times$ factor at ambient temperature

$= volume_{ATPS} \times$ Factor at 25 °C

$= 600 \times 1.075$ (Appendix E)

$= 645$ mL

## EXERCISE 1

A tidal volume was recorded at 23 °C. What should be the factor for converting this measurement from ATPS to BTPS at normal body temperature (37 °C)?

[Answer: Conversion factor = 1.085]

## EXERCISE 2

A peak flow of 120 L / min was recorded at 27 °C. What is the corrected flow rate at body temperature (37 °C)?

[Answer: Flow rate = 127.56 or 128 L / min]

| **REFERENCE**   Scanlan

# SELF-ASSESSMENT QUESTIONS

7a.   The vital capacity (*VC*) measured under ATPS conditions is 3600 mL. What is the corrected *VC* at BTPS if the measurement was done at 27 ˚C? (Conversion factor from 27 to 37 ˚C is 1.063.)

(A) 360 mL

(B) 3000 mL

(C) 3387 mL

(D) 3600 mL

(E) 3827 mL

7b.   An average tidal volume ($V_T$) of 580 mL was recorded under ATPS conditions. If the ambient temperature at the time of measurement is 25 ˚C, what should be the factor for converting this volume from ATPS to BTPS (Appendix E)? What is the corrected $V_T$ under BTPS conditions?

(A) 1.080; 540 mL

(B) 1.080; 580 mL

(C) 1.075; 624 mL

(D) 1.075; 780 mL

(E) 1.068; 851 mL

# 8

# Bicarbonate Corrections of Base Deficit

## NOTES

This equation calculates the amount of sodium bicarbonate needed to correct severe metabolic acidosis. The value $\frac{1}{4}$ in the equation represents the amount of extracellular water in the body ($\frac{1}{3}$ has been used as an alternative factor to estimate the amount of extracellular fluid).

During cardiopulmonary resuscitation or when the patient's perfusion is unsatisfactory, the entire calculated amount is given.

If cardiac massage is not required, half of the calculated dose is given initially to prevent overcompensation. Bicarbonate may not be needed when the arterial pH is greater than 7.20 or the base deficit is less than 10 mEq/L. For patients with diabetic ketoacidosis, bicarbonate may best be withheld until the pH is less than 7.10.

According to the *Textbook of Advanced Cardiac Life Support* by AHA, use of bicarbonate in cardiopulmonary resuscitation is not recommended. However, in severe, pre-existing metabolic acidosis, 1 mEq/kg of sodium bicarbonate may be used; subsequent doses should not exceed 0.5 mEq/kg. Refer to the current edition of the *ACLS* textbook for specific indications.

## EQUATION

$$HCO_3^- = \frac{(BD \times kg)}{4}$$

$HCO_3^-$:  Sodium bicarbonate needed to correct severe base deficit, in mEq/L

BD  :  Base deficit in mEq/L, negative base excess (–BE)

kg  :  Body weight in kilograms

## EXAMPLE

How many mEq/L of bicarbonate are needed to correct a base deficit of 12 mEq/L if the patient's body weight is 60 kg? If the initial dose is $\frac{1}{2}$ of the calculated amount, what is the initial dose?

$$HCO_3^- = \frac{(BD \times kg)}{4}$$

$$= \frac{(12 \times 60)}{4}$$

$$= \frac{(720)}{4}$$

$$= 180 \text{ mEq/L}$$

Initial dose $= \frac{1}{2} \times 180$ or 90 mEq/L

## EXERCISE

Calculate the amount of bicarbonate for a 70-kg patient whose BE is –18 mEq/L. What is the initial dose?

[Answer: $HCO_3^-$ = 315 mEq/L; initial dose = 158 mEq/L]

## REFERENCES

Grauer; Malley; McIntyre; Shapiro (1)

## SELF-ASSESSMENT QUESTIONS

8a.   A 53-kg patient has a base deficit of 30 mEq/L. If indicated, the initial amount of bicarbonate needed for this patient is about:

(A) bicarbonate is not indicated

(B) 265 mEq/L

(C) 199 mEq/L

(D) 133 mEq/L

(E) 100 mEq/L

8b.   Calculate the amount of bicarbonate needed to correct a base deficit of 20 mEq/L for a patient weighing 80 kg. If the initial dose is $\frac{1}{2}$ of the calculated amount, what should be the initial dose?

(A) 800 mEq/L; initial dose = 400 mEq/L

(B) 400 mEq/L; initial dose = 200 mEq/L

(C) 200 mEq/L; initial dose = 100 mEq/L

(D) 80 mEq/L; initial dose = 40 mEq/L

(E) 20 mEq/L; initial dose = 10 mEq/L

8c.   How much bicarbonate is needed to correct a base deficit of 16 mEq/L for a patient whose body weight is 70 kg? What should be the initial dose if half of the calculated amount is needed?

(A) 16 mEq/L; initial dose = 8 mEq/L

(B) 150 mEq/L; initial dose = 75 mEq/L

(C) 180 mEq/L; initial dose = 90 mEq/L

(D) 220 mEq/L; initial dose = 110 mEq/L

(E) 280 mEq/L; initial dose = 140 mEq/L

# CHAPTER

# 9
# Body Surface Area

The body surface area (*BSA*) is used to calculate the cardiac index, the stroke volume index, or the drug dosages for adults and children. One way to find the body surface area is to use the DuBois Body Surface Chart (Appendix F). If the chart is not available, this BSA equation can be used.

To use the equation, the patient's body weight in *kilograms* must be known.

Divide the body weight in pounds by 2.2 to get kilograms.

## EQUATION

$$BSA = \frac{(4 \times kg) + 7}{kg + 90}$$

$BSA$  :  Body surface area in $m^2$
$kg$   :  Body weight in kilograms

## NORMAL VALUE

Adult average $BSA = 1.7\ m^2$

## EXAMPLE

What is the calculated body surface area of a child weighing 44 pounds?

$$44\ lbs = \frac{44}{2.2}\ kg$$

$$= 20\ kg$$

$$BSA = \frac{(4 \times kg) + 7}{kg + 90}$$

$$= \frac{(4 \times 20) + 7}{20 + 90}$$

$$= \frac{80 + 7}{110}$$

$$= \frac{87}{110}$$

$$= 0.79\ m^2$$

## EXERCISE 1

Calculate the body surface area of a 132-lb patient.

[Answer: $BSA = 1.65\ m^2$]

**EXERCISE 2**    Use the DuBois Body Surface Chart in Appendix F to find the body surface area of a person who is 5′ 6″ and 140 lb. Using the equation and weight provided, calculate the body surface area.

[Answer: *BSA* (chart) = 1.72 m$^2$; *BSA* (calculated) = 1.70 m$^2$]

**REFERENCE**    Hegstad

**SEE**    *Appendix F, DuBois Body Surface Chart.*

## SELF-ASSESSMENT QUESTIONS

9a.    Calculate the body surface area (BSA) of a person weighing 80 kg. Given: BSA = $\dfrac{(4 \times kg) + 7}{kg + 90}$.

(A) 1.92 kg

(B) 1.92 m

(C) 1.92 m$^2$

(D) 4.36 ft$^2$

(E) 4.36 ft$^3$

9b.    What is the calculated body surface area (BSA) of a person weighing 120 lb? (2.2 lb = 1 kg.) If the same person is 5 ft 5 in. tall, what is the body surface area using the DuBois Body Surface Chart (Appendix F)?

(A) 1.56 m$^2$; 1.59 m$^2$

(B) 1.76 m$^2$; 1.59 m$^2$

(C) 1.89 m$^2$; 1.66 m$^2$

(D) 1.93 m$^2$; 1.66 m$^2$

(E) 2.04 m$^2$; 1.85 m$^2$

# CHAPTER

# *10*
# Cardiac Index (*CI* )

## NOTES

Normal cardiac output for a resting adult ranges from 4 to 8 L/min.

Cardiac index (*CI* ) is used to normalize cardiac output measurements among patients of varying body size. For instance, a cardiac output of 4 L/min may be normal for an average-sized person but low for a large-sized person. The cardiac index will be able to distinguish this difference based on body size.

*CI* values between 1.8 and 2.5 L/min/m$^2$ indicate hypoperfusion. Values less than 1.8 may be indicative of cardiogenic shock.

## EQUATION

$$CI = \frac{CO}{BSA}$$

$CI$ : Cardiac index in L/min/m$^2$
$CO$ : Cardiac output in L/min ($Q_T$)
$BSA$ : Body surface area in m$^2$ *

## NORMAL VALUE

2.5 to 3.5 L/min/m$^2$

## EXAMPLE

Given: Cardiac output $= 4$ L/min
Body surface area $= 1.4$ m$^2$
Calculate the cardiac index.

$$CI = \frac{CO}{BSA}$$
$$= \frac{4}{1.4}$$
$$= 2.86 \text{ L/min/m}^2$$

## EXERCISE

Given: Cardiac output $= 4$ L/min
Body surface area $= 2.5$ m$^2$
Find the cardiac index (*CI*).

[Answer: $CI = 1.6$ L/min/m$^2$]

## REFERENCES

Bustin; Des Jardins

## SEE

*Appendix F, DuBois Body Surface Chart; Appendix G, Hemodynamic Normal Ranges.*

*Chapter 9 Body Surface Area*

# Self-Assessment Questions

10a. Given: Cardiac output = 4.5 L/min, body surface area = 1.0 m$^2$. What is the calculated cardiac index?

(A) 0.22 m$^2$/L/min

(B) 3.5 L/min/m$^2$

(C) 4.5 L/min/m$^2$

(D) 4.5 m$^2$/L/min

(E) 5.5 L/min/m$^2$

10b. Given the following measurements from a patient in the coronary intensive care unit: cardiac output = 5 L/min, body surface area = 1.7 m$^2$. What is the patient's cardiac index? Is it normal for this patient?

(A) 2.94 L/min/m$^2$; abnormal

(B) 2.94 L/min/m$^2$; normal

(C) 3.3 L/min/m$^2$; abnormal

(D) 3.3 L/min/m$^2$; normal

(E) 8.5 L/min/m$^2$; abnormal

10c. An 85-kg patient has the following measurements: cardiac output = 5 L/min, body surface area = 2.9 m$^2$. What is the calculated cardiac index? Is it normal for this patient?

(A) 1.72 L/min/m$^2$; abnormal

(B) 1.72 L/min/m$^2$; normal

(C) 2.1 L/min; abnormal

(D) 14.5 L/min/m$^2$; normal

(E) 14.5 L/min/m$^2$; abnormal

10d. The following measurements are obtained from a patient whose admitting diagnosis is Pickwickian syndrome with sleep apnea: cardiac output ($CO$) = 6 L/min, body surface area = 3.3 m$^2$. Is the patient's cardiac output within the normal range? Is the cardiac index ($CI$) normal?

(A) $CO$ within normal range; $CI$ abnormal

(B) $CO$ and $CI$ within normal range

(C) $CO$ abnormal; $CI$ within normal range

(D) $CO$ and $CI$ abnormal

(E) insufficient information to compute answer

10e. The following values are obtained from a 50-year-old patient with congestive heart failure: cardiac output = 3.0 L/min, body surface area = 1.0 m$^2$. Is the patient's cardiac output ($CO$) normal? Cardiac index ($CI$)?

(A) $CO$ within normal range; $CI$ abnormal

(B) $CO$ and $CI$ within normal range

(C) $CO$ abnormal; $CI$ within normal range

(D) $CO$ and $CI$ abnormal

(E) Questionable data. Repeat measurements required.

10f. Ms. Morgan, a 68-year-old postsurgical patient, has a cardiac output of 4.9 L/min. If her estimated body surface area is 1.4 m$^2$, what is her cardiac index? Is it within the normal range?

(A) 6.9 L/min/m$^2$; normal

(B) 6.9 L/min/m$^2$; abnormal

(C) 4.1 L/min/m$^2$; normal

(D) 4.1 L/min/m$^2$; abnormal

(E) 3.5 L/min/m$^2$; normal

CO  4.8

6' feet

180#

2.1

CHAPTER

# 11
# Cardiac Output (*CO*): Fick's Estimated Method

**EQUATION 1**

$$CO = \frac{O_2 \text{ consumption}}{C_aO_2 - C_{\bar{v}}O_2}$$

**EQUATION 2**

$$CO = \frac{130 \times BSA}{C_aO_2 - C_{\bar{v}}O_2}$$

$CO$ : Cardiac output in L/min ($Q_T$)

$O_2$ consumption : Estimated to be $130 \times BSA$, in mL/min ($\dot{V}O_2$)

$C_aO_2$ : Arterial oxygen content in vol%

$C_{\bar{v}}O_2$ : Mixed venous oxygen content in vol%

130 : Estimated $O_2$ consumption rate of an adult, in mL/min/m$^2$

$BSA$: Body surface area in m$^2$

**NORMAL VALUE**

$CO = 4$ to $8$ L/min

**EXAMPLE**

Given: Body surface area = 1.6 m$^2$
Arterial $O_2$ content = 20 vol%
Mixed venous $O_2$ content = 15 vol%

$$CO = \frac{O_2 \text{ consumption}}{C_aO_2 - C_{\bar{v}}O_2}$$

$$= \frac{130 \times BSA}{C_aO_2 - C_{\bar{v}}O_2}$$

$$= \frac{130 \times 1.6}{20\% - 15\%}$$

$$= \frac{208}{5\%}$$

$$= \frac{208}{0.05}$$

$$= 4160 \text{ mL/min or } 4.16 \text{ L/min}$$

**EXERCISE**

Given: $BSA = 1.2 \text{ m}^2$

$C_aO_2 = 19 \text{ vol}\%$

$C_{\bar{v}}O_2 = 14 \text{ vol}\%$

Calculate the cardiac output using Fick's estimated method.

[Answer: $CO = 3120 \text{ mL/min}$ or $3.12 \text{ L/min}$]

**REFERENCE**

Bustin

**SEE**

*Oxygen Consumption ($\dot{V}O_2$); Oxygen Content, Arterial ($C_aO_2$); Oxygen Content, Mixed Venous ($C_{\bar{v}}O_2$); Appendix F, DuBois Body Surface Chart; Appendix G, Hemodynamic Normal Ranges.*

## Self-Assessment Questions

11a. Since oxygen consumption in mL/min can be estimated by using the formula 130 mL/min/m² × BSA m², what is the estimated $O_2$ consumption for a patient whose body surface area (BSA) is $1.5 \text{ m}^2$?

(A) 87 mL/min

(B) 100 mL/min

(C) 130 mL/min

(D) 150 mL/min

(E) 195 mL/min

11b. Given: oxygen consumption ($\dot{V}O_2$) = 156 mL, arterial $O_2$ content ($C_aO_2$) = 19 vol%, mixed venous $O_2$ content ($C_{\bar{v}}O_2$) = 15 vol%. Calculate the cardiac output using Fick's estimated method.

(A) 156 mL/min

(B) 892 mL/min

(C) 2.3 L/min

(D) 3.9 L/min

(E) 4.8 L/min

11c. The following hemodynamic values are obtained from a patient in the intensive care unit: estimated oxygen consumption ($\dot{V}O_2$) = 180 mL, arterial $O_2$ content ($C_aO_2$) = 18.4 vol%, mixed venous $O_2$ content ($C_{\bar{v}}O_2$) = 14.4 vol%. Calculate the cardiac output using Fick's estimated method. Is it normal?

(A) 4.5 L/min; normal

(B) 5.5 L/min; normal

(C) 6 L/min; normal

(D) 6.5 L/min; abnormal

(E) 7.5 L/min; abnormal

11d. A patient whose body surface area is about 1.4 m$^2$ has the following oxygen content values: $C_aO_2$ = 19.5 vol%, $C_{\bar{v}}O_2$ = 14.5 vol%. What is the cardiac output based on Fick's estimated method?

(A) 182 mL/min

(B) 980 mL/min

(C) 2.73 L/min

(D) 2.98 L/min

(E) 3.64 L/min

# CHAPTER

# *12*

# Compliance: Dynamic ($C_{dyn}$)

## NOTES

Dynamic compliance is used to assess changes in the non-elastic (airway) resistance to air flow.

When the dynamic compliance changes *independently*, without corresponding change in static compliance, it is indicative of airway resistance changes. For example, if the dynamic compliance decreases with minimal or no decrease in static compliance, it is likely caused by an increase in nonelastic (airway) resistance. This type of resistance change may include bronchospasm, main-stem intubation, kinked tubing or endotracheal tube, mucus plugs, etc.

Figure 2 shows the relative positions of static and dynamic compliance curves. Figure 3 illustrates the use of dynamic and static compliance measurements for interpretation of changes in nonelastic (airway) resistance.

## EQUATION

$$C_{dyn} = \frac{\Delta V}{\Delta P}$$

$C_{dyn}$ : Dynamic compliance in mL / cm $H_2O$

$\Delta V$ : Corrected tidal volume in mL

$\Delta P$ : Pressure change (Peak airway pressure – PEEP) in cm $H_2O$

## NORMAL VALUE

30 to 40 mL / cm $H_2O$

If the patient is intubated, use serial measurements to establish trend.

## EXAMPLE

Given: $\Delta V$                       = 500 mL

       Peak airway pressure    = 30 cm $H_2O$

       PEEP                    = 10 cm $H_2O$

Calculate the dynamic compliance.

$$C_{dyn} = \frac{\Delta V}{\Delta P}$$

$$= \frac{500}{30 - 10}$$

$$= \frac{500}{20}$$

$$= 25 \text{ mL/cm } H_2O$$

## EXERCISE

Given: Corrected tidal volume  = 800 mL

       Peak airway pressure    = 40 cm $H_2O$

       PEEP                    = 5 cm $H_2O$

Calculate the dynamic compliance.

[Answer: $C_{dyn}$ = 22.9 or 23 mL / cm $H_2O$]

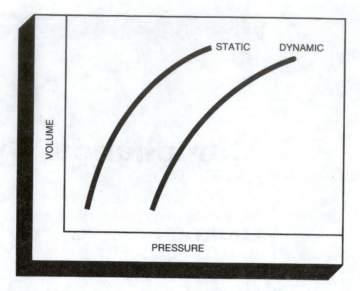

**Figure 2** *Relative positions of static and dynamic compliance curves. Each curve consists of a series of volume/pressure measurements. Shifting of the curve(s) to the left indicates increase of compliance, whereas shifting of the curve(s) to the right means decrease of compliance. The dynamic compliance curve can shift independently. However, any shifting of the static compliance curve is always accompanied by a similar shift of the dynamic compliance curve.*

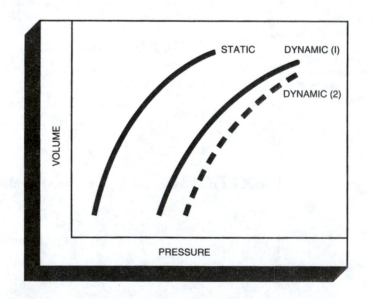

**Figure 3** *Shifting of the dynamic compliance curve. The dynamic compliance curve shifts to the right with a decrease in dynamic compliance (increase in nonelastic or airway resistance). Note that shifting of the dynamic compliance curve occurs independently [dynamic (2)], and the position of the static compliance curve is unchanged. Improvement of the nonelastic or airway resistance to a normal state will cause the dynamic compliance curve to return to its original position [dynamic (1)].*

**REFERENCES**   Barnes, Kacmarek

*See Corrected Tidal Volume ($V_T$); Compliance: Static ($C_{st}$).*

## Self-Assessment Questions

**12a.** Given: corrected tidal volume = 760 mL, peak airway pressure = 38 cm $H_2O$. Calculate the dynamic compliance.

(A) 10 mL/cm $H_2O$

(B) 15 mL/cm $H_2O$

(C) 20 mL/cm $H_2O$

(D) 25 mL/cm $H_2O$

(E) 30 mL/cm $H_2O$

**12b.** What is the patient's dynamic compliance if the corrected tidal volume = 800 mL, peak airway pressure = 45 cm $H_2O$, and PEEP = 15 cm $H_2O$?

(A) 17.8 mL/cm $H_2O$

(B) 20.5 mL/cm $H_2O$

(C) 26.7 mL/cm $H_2O$

(D) 41.1 mL/cm $H_2O$

(E) 53.3 mL/cm $H_2O$

**12c.** A patient who is on a volume ventilator has the following measurements: corrected tidal volume = 780 mL, peak airway pressure = 55 cm $H_2O$, plateau pressure = 35 cm $H_2O$, and PEEP = 10 cm $H_2O$. What is the dynamic compliance?

(A) 78 mL/cm $H_2O$

(B) 31.2 mL/cm $H_2O$

(C) 22.3 mL/cm $H_2O$

(D) 17.3 mL/cm $H_2O$

(E) 14.2 mL/cm $H_2O$

**12d.** If a patient's corrected tidal volume is 800 mL and the corresponding peak airway pressure is 20 cm $H_2O$, what is the calculated dynamic compliance?

(A) 16 mL/cm $H_2O$

(B) 20 mL/cm $H_2O$

(C) 25 mL/cm $H_2O$

(D) 40 mL/cm $H_2O$

(E) 80 mL/cm $H_2O$

# CHAPTER

# *13*
# Compliance: Static (*C*st)

Static compliance is used to assess changes of the elastic (lung parenchymal) resistance to air flow.

The static compliance causes the dynamic compliance to increase or decrease correspondingly, and by similar proportion.

When the static and dynamic compliances decrease in the same proportion, it is indicative of an increase of elastic (lung parenchymal) resistance such as pneumonia or pulmonary edema. On the other hand, improvement of any lung parenchymal disease would increase the static *and* the dynamic compliance.

Figure 2 (p. 36) shows the relative positions of static and dynamic compliance curves. Figure 4 illustrates the use of dynamic and static compliance measurements for interpretation of changes in elastic (lung parenchymal) resistance.

## EQUATION

$$C_{st} = \frac{\Delta V}{\Delta P}$$

$C_{st}$ : Static compliance in mL / cm $H_2O$

$\Delta V$ : Corrected tidal volume in mL

$\Delta P$ : Pressure change (Plateau pressure – PEEP) in cm $H_2O$

## NORMAL VALUE

40 to 60 mL / cm $H_2O$

If the patient is intubated, use serial measurements to establish trend.

## EXAMPLE

Given: $\Delta V$ = 500 mL

Plateau pressure = 20 cm $H_2O$

PEEP = 5 cm $H_2O$

Calculate the static compliance:

$$C_{st} = \frac{\Delta V}{\Delta P}$$

$$= \frac{500}{20 - 5}$$

$$= \frac{500}{15}$$

= 33.3 or 33 mL/cm $H_2O$

## EXERCISE

Given: Corrected tidal volume = 800 mL

Plateau pressure = 35 cm $H_2O$

PEEP = 5 cm $H_2O$

Calculate the static compliance.

[Answer: $C_{st}$ = 26.7 or 27 mL / cm $H_2O$]

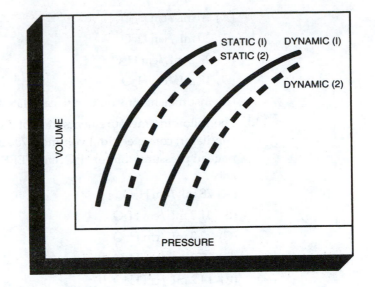

**Figure 4** *Shifting of the dynamic and static compliance curves. Both curves shift to the right with a decrease in static compliance (increase in elastic or lung parenchymal resistance). Note that the static and dynamic compliance curves are both shifted to the right [static (2) and dynamic (2)]. Improvement of the elastic or lung parenchymal resistance to a normal state will cause both of the compliance curves to return to their original positions [static (1) and dynamic (1)].*

### REFERENCES    Barnes, Kacmarek

*See Corrected Tidal Volume ($V_T$); Compliance: Dynamic ($C_{dyn}$).*

## *Self-Assessment Questions*

13a. $\dfrac{Corrected\ tidal\ volume}{plateau\ pressure}$ is equal to:

   (A) static compliance

   (B) dynamic compliance

   (C) airway resistance

   (D) airway conductance

   (E) pulmonary elastance

13b. Given the following ventilation parameters: corrected tidal volume = 700 mL, plateau pressure = 30 cm $H_2O$. Calculate the static compliance.

   (A) 7 mL / cm $H_2O$

   (B) 10 mL / cm $H_2O$

   (C) 20.8 mL / cm $H_2O$

   (D) 23.3 mL / cm $H_2O$

   (E) 70 mL / cm $H_2O$

13c. Calculate a patient's static compliance given the following ventilation measurements: corrected tidal volume = 900 mL, plateau pressure = 40 cm $H_2O$, and PEEP = 10 cm $H_2O$.

(A) 90 mL / cm $H_2O$

(B) 30 mL / cm $H_2O$

(C) 22.5 mL / cm $H_2O$

(D) 18 mL / cm $H_2O$

(E) insufficient information to calculate answer

13d. The following measurements are obtained from a patient who is on a volume ventilator: corrected tidal volume = 780 mL, peak airway pressure = 55 cm $H_2O$, plateau pressure = 35 cm $H_2O$, and PEEP = 10 cm $H_2O$. What is the static compliance?

(A) 78 mL / cm $H_2O$

(B) 31.2 mL / cm $H_2O$

(C) 22.3 mL / cm $H_2O$

(D) 17.3 mL / cm $H_2O$

(E) 14.2 mL / cm $H_2O$

13e. Five sets of values have been obtained to determine the optimum PEEP, based on the best static compliance. Which of the following measurements indicates the best static compliance?

| | Corrected Tidal Volume | Plateau Pressure | PEEP |
|---|---|---|---|
| (A) | 750 mL | 30 cm $H_2O$ | 8 cm $H_2O$ |
| (B) | 775 mL | 31 cm $H_2O$ | 10 cm $H_2O$ |
| (C) | 790 mL | 32 cm $H_2O$ | 12 cm $H_2O$ |
| (D) | 795 mL | 36 cm $H_2O$ | 14 cm $H_2O$ |
| (E) | 800 mL | 38 cm $H_2O$ | 16 cm $H_2O$ |

# CHAPTER

# *14*

# Compliance: Total ($C_T$)

**EQUATION**

$$\frac{1}{C_T} = \frac{1}{C_L} + \frac{1}{C_{CW}}$$

$\dfrac{1}{C_T}$ : Reciprocal of total compliance (lung and chest wall)

$\dfrac{1}{C_L}$ : Reciprocal of lung compliance

$\dfrac{1}{C_{CW}}$ : Reciprocal of chest-wall compliance

This equation describes the relationship among total compliance, lung compliance, and chest-wall compliance. It is essential to note that the *reciprocals* of these values are related. For example, if the lung and chest-wall compliance values are both 0.2 L/cm $H_2O$, the sum of these two reciprocals (total compliance) is 0.1 L/cm $H_2O$.

$$\frac{1}{0.2} + \frac{1}{0.2} = \frac{(1+1)}{0.2}$$

$$= \frac{2}{0.2}$$

$$= \frac{1}{0.1}$$

With an intact lung-thorax system, the lung compliance equals the chest-wall compliance. When this condition exists, the total compliance is half of the lung compliance or chest-wall compliance.

**REFERENCE**   Wojciechowski

## *Self-Assessment Questions*

14a. Which of the following groups of compliance values equal one another in an intact lung-thorax system?
(A) lung compliance and chest-wall compliance
(B) total compliance and chest-wall compliance

(C)  total compliance and lung compliance

(D)  total compliance, lung compliance, and chest-wall compliance

(E)  none of the above

14b.  Total compliance is about _____ L/cm $H_2O$, _____ the normal lung compliance value.

(A) 0.1; twice

(B) 0.1; half of

(C) 0.2; twice

(D) 0.2; half of

(E) 0.2; same as

14c.  The normal chest-wall compliance is about _____ L/cm $H_2O$, _____ the normal lung compliance value.

(A) 0.1; twice

(B) 0.1; half of

(C) 0.2; twice

(D) 0.2; half of

(E) 0.2; same as

14d.  Under normal conditions, all of the following statements are true *except*:

(A) Chest-wall compliance is same as lung compliance.

(B) Chest-wall compliance is greater than total compliance.

(C) Lung compliance is greater than total compliance.

(D) The sum of lung and chest wall compliance is greater than total compliance.

(E) Total compliance has the lowest value of all three compliances.

# CHAPTER

# 15

# Corrected Tidal Volume ($V_T$)

*NOTE*

The tubing compression factor on a volume-limited ventilator can be determined by the following procedures: (1) Set the respiratory rate at 10 to 16/min and the tidal volume between 100 and 200 mL with minimum flow rate and maximum pressure limit; (2) completely occlude the patient Y-connection of the ventilator circuit; (3) record the observed expired volume (mL) and the peak inspiratory pressure (cm $H_2O$); and (4) divide the observed expired volume by the peak inspiratory pressure. The result will be the tubing compression factor in mL/cm $H_2O$.

## EQUATION

Corrected $V_T$ = Expired $V_T$ – Tubing Volume

Expired $V_T$  :  Expired tidal volume in mL
Tubing volume :  Volume "lost" in tubing during inspiratory phase (Pressure change × 3 mL/cm $H_2O$)*

## EXAMPLE

| | |
|---|---|
| Expired $V_T$ | = 650 mL |
| Peak airway pressure | = 25 cm $H_2O$ |
| Positive end-expiratory pressure (PEEP) | = 5 cm $H_2O$ |
| Tubing compression factor | = 3 mL/cm $H_2O$* |

Calculate the corrected tidal volume.

Because

Tubing volume = Pressure change × 3 mL/cm $H_2O$
$\qquad$ = (25 – 5) cm $H_2O$ × 3 mL/cm $H_2O$
$\qquad$ = 20 × 3 mL
$\qquad$ = 60 mL

then

Corrected $V_T$ = Expired $V_T$ – Tubing Volume
$\qquad$ = 650 – 60
$\qquad$ = 590 mL

## EXERCISE

| | |
|---|---|
| Expired $V_T$ | = 780 mL |
| Peak airway pressure | = 45 cm $H_2O$ |
| PEEP | = 10 cm $H_2O$ |
| Tubing compression factor | = 3 mL/cm $H_2O$ |

Calculate the corrected tidal volume.

[Answer: Corrected $V_T$ = 675 mL]

## REFERENCES

Barnes, Scanlan

*The tubing compression factor ranges from 1 to 8 mL/cm $H_2O$. This factor may change according to (1) the type of ventilator used, (2) the type of circuit used, and (3) the water level in the humidifier.*

## Self-Assessment Questions

15a. What is the tubing compression volume if the tubing compression factor is 3 mL/cm $H_2O$ and the pressure change is 30 cm $H_2O$?

(A) 3 mL

(B) 30 mL

(C) 33 mL

(D) 60 mL

(E) 90 mL

15b. The information below is obtained from a routine ventilator check. Calculate the corrected tidal volume.

$$\begin{aligned}
\text{Expired } V_T &= 780 \text{ mL} \\
\text{Peak airway pressure} &= 45 \text{ cm } H_2O \\
\text{Positive end-expiratory pressure (PEEP)} &= 5 \text{ cm } H_2O \\
\text{Tubing compression factor} &= 3 \text{ mL/cm } H_2O
\end{aligned}$$

(A) 645 mL

(B) 660 mL

(C) 765 mL

(D) 780 mL

(E) 900 mL

15c. Calculate the corrected tidal volume with the following information obtained during a ventilator check:

$$\begin{aligned}
\text{Expired } V_T &= 780 \text{ mL} \\
\text{Peak airway pressure} &= 45 \text{ cm } H_2O \\
\text{Positive end-expiratory pressure (PEEP)} &= 5 \text{ cm } H_2O \\
\text{Tubing compression factor} &= 5 \text{ mL/cm } H_2O
\end{aligned}$$

(A) 555 mL

(B) 580 mL

(C) 620 mL

(D) 755 mL

(E) 780 mL

# CHAPTER

# *16*
# Correction Factor

## NOTES

**Example 1**

In this example, the expected pressure is the barometric pressure, 1000 cm $H_2O$ or 735 mm Hg. During inspiration the circuit pressure is 50 cm $H_2O$ higher than the barometric pressure. The measured pressure is therefore 1050 cm $H_2O$ (1000 + 50). The correction factor 0.952 is used to multiply the $F_IO_2$ as recorded by the analyzer. For example, if the oxygen analyzer reads 60%, the corrected $F_IO_2$ becomes 57% (60% x 0.952 = 57.12%).

**Example 2**

In the first part of Example 2, the measured volume is greater than the expected volume during calibration. The correction factor is therefore less than 1. Once a correction factor is obtained, subsequent measurements may be "corrected" by multiplying them by this correction factor. For example, if the correction factor is 0.993 and the spirometer reads a tidal volume of 600 mL, the corrected tidal volume becomes 596 mL (600 x 0.993 = 595.8 mL).

In the second part of Example 2, the measured volume is smaller than the expected volume during calibration. The correction factor is therefore greater than 1. For example, if the correction factor is 1.014 and the spirometer reads a tidal volume of 600 mL, the corrected tidal volume becomes 608 mL (600 x 1.014 = 608.4 mL).

## EQUATION

$$\text{Correction Factor} = \frac{\text{Expected}}{\text{Measured}}$$

Expected : Expected (input) measurements such as barometric pressure, volume in calibration syringe

Measured : Actual (output) measurements such as pressure in ventilator circuit, volume recorded by spirometry

## NORMAL VALUE

Correction factor > 1 if expected > measured.
Correction factor not needed if expected = measured.
Corrected factor < 1 if expected < measured.

## EXAMPLE 1

A galvanic cell oxygen analyzer is being used in a ventilator circuit (circuit pressure = 50 cm $H_2O$). If barometric pressure is 735 mmHg (1000 cm $H_2O$), what should be the correction factor for subsequent $F_IO_2$ measurements?

$$\text{Correction factor} = \frac{\text{Expected}}{\text{Measure}}$$
$$= \frac{1000}{1000 + 50}$$
$$= \frac{1000}{1050}$$
$$= 0.952$$

## EXAMPLE 2

A 3-L calibration syringe is used to calibrate the pulmonary function spirometer. If the spirometer records a volume of 3.02 L, what should be the correction factor for subsequent volume measurements?

$$\text{Correction factor} = \frac{\text{Expected}}{\text{Measured}}$$
$$= \frac{3.00}{3.02}$$
$$= 0.993$$

What should be the correction factor if the spirometer records a volume of 2.96 L?

$$\text{Correction factor} = \frac{\text{Expected}}{\text{Measured}}$$

$$= \frac{3.00}{2.96}$$

$$= 1.014$$

**EXERCISE 1**

A polarographic oxygen analyzer is being used in a ventilator circuit (circuit pressure = 45 cm $H_2O$). If barometric pressure is 996 cm $H_2O$, what should be the correction factor for all subsequent $F_IO_2$ measurements?

[Answer: Correction factor = 0.957]

**EXERCISE 2**

A 3-L calibration syringe is used to calibrate the pulmonary function spirometer. If the spirometer records a volume of 2.88 L, what should be the correction factor for subsequent volume measurements?

[Answer: Correction factor = 1.042]

What should be the correction factor if the spirometer records a volume of 3.07 L?

[Answer: Correction factor = 0.977]

**REFERENCES**

Madama; Ruppel

*See Pressure Conversions in Section 6 to convert pressures from mm Hg to cm $H_2O$.*

# Self-Assessment Questions

16a. The correction factor used in calibration of a pulmonary function spirometer or other similar device can be calculated by using the following solution:

(A) Expected value + Actual value

(B) Expected value − Actual value

(C) Expected value × Actual value

(D) $\dfrac{\text{Expected value}}{\text{Actual value}}$

(E) $\dfrac{\text{Expected value} + \text{Actual value}}{\text{Actual value}}$

16b. Exactly 3 L of air from a calibration syringe is used to calibrate the pulmonary function spirometer. The recorded volume is 2.89 L. Calculate the correction factor for subsequent volume measurements made by this spirometer.

(A) 0.926

(B) 0.963

(C) 1.038

(D) 1.045

(E) 1.073

16c. A known flow rate at precisely 4 L/sec is introduced into the spirometer, and the spirometer records a flow rate of 4.07 L/sec. What should be the correction factor for subsequent flow rate measurements?

(A) 0.946

(B) 0.953

(C) 0.970

(D) 0.983

(E) 1.017

16d. If the correction factor for a spirometer is 0.993 and the spirometer measures a vital capacity of 3.8 L, what should be the corrected vital capacity?

(A) 3.56 L

(B) 3.62 L

(C) 3.77 L

(D) 3.88 L

(E) 3.97 L

16e. A polarographic oxygen analyzer is being used in a ventilator circuit (circuit pressure = 45 cm $H_2O$). If barometric pressure is 900 cm $H_2O$, what should be the correction factor for all subsequent $F_IO_2$ measurements?

(A) 0.900

(B) 0.919

(C) 0.921

(D) 0.934

(E) 0.952

16f. A pressure-sensitive oxygen analyzer (galvanic cell) is used to measure the $F_IO_2$ in a ventilator circuit. Calculate the correction factor for the $F_IO_2$ measurements if the barometric pressure is 1003 cm $H_2O$ and the circuit pressure is 60 cm $H_2O$ over the barometric pressure.

(A) 0.911

(B) 0.944

(C) 0.965

(D) 1.003

(E) 1.033

16g. The sensor of a galvanic cell oxygen analyzer is placed in-line of a ventilator circuit. An $F_IO_2$ reading of 60% is obtained. What is the corrected $F_IO_2$ if the correction factor is 0.934 for this oxygen analyzer?

(A) 56%

(B) 60%

(C) 62%

(D) 65%

(E) 68%

# *17*
# Dalton's Law
# of Partial Pressure

## NOTES

Dalton's law, named for the English chemist John Dalton (1766-1844), states that the total pressure exerted by a gas mixture is equal to the sum of the partial pressures of all gases in the mixture. Water vapor is considered a gas, and it exerts water vapor pressure. Table 3 shows the gases that compose the barometric pressure in the absence of water vapor.

Under unusual atmospheric environments, individual gas pressures increase in hyperbaric conditions (e.g., hyperbaric chamber, under water) and decrease in hypobaric conditions (e.g., high altitude) according to the percentage of the total volume each gas occupies.

## EQUATION

Total pressure = $P_1 + P_2 + P_3 + ...$

| | | |
|---|---|---|
| Total pressure | : | Pressure of all gases in mixture |
| $P_1$ | : | Pressure of gas 1 in gas mixture |
| $P_2$ | : | Pressure of gas 2 in gas mixture |
| $P_3$ | : | Pressure of gas 3 in gas mixture |
| ... | : | All other gases |

**Table 3.    Gases That Compose the Barometric Pressure**

| GAS | % OF ATMOSPHERE | PARTIAL PRESSURE OF DRY GAS (mm Hg) |
|---|---|---|
| Nitrogen ($N_2$) | 78.08 | 593 |
| Oxygen ($O_2$) | 20.95 | 159 |
| Argon (Ar) | 0.93 | 7 |
| Carbon Dioxide ($CO_2$) | 0.03 | 0.2 |

From Des Jardins, T.R., *Cardiopulmonary Anatomy and Physiology: Essentials for Respiratory Care*, 3rd ed. Albany, NY: Delmar Publishers, 1998.

## REFERENCES    Des Jardins; Scanlan

## SEE    *Partial Pressure of a Dry Gas.*

## Self-Assessment Questions

17a.  The sum of partial pressures exerted by all gases in the atmosphere equals the barometric pressure. This is a statement of

(A) Dalton's law

(B) Henry's law

(C) Charles' law

(D) Graham's law

(E)  Hooke's law

17b.  If the $PO_2$ is 100 mm Hg at one barometric pressure (760 mm Hg), what is the approximate $PO_2$ if the pressure is increased to 1520 mm Hg in a hyperbaric chamber?

(A) 25 mm Hg

(B)  50 mm Hg

(C)  100 mm Hg

(D) 200 mm Hg

(E)  insufficient information to compute answer

17c.  The normal predicted $PO_2$ in an area 10,000 ft above sea level should be _____ that at sea level because of the _____ condition at high altitude.

(A)  the same as; hyperbaric

(B)  higher than; hyperbaric

(C)  higher than; hypobaric

(D)  lower than; hyperbaric

(E)  lower than; hypobaric

# CHAPTER

# *18*

# Deadspace to Tidal Volume Ratio ($V_D/V_T$)

## NOTES

$\frac{V_D}{V_T}$ ratio is used to approximate the portion of tidal volume not taking part in gas exchange (i.e., wasted ventilation). A large $\frac{V_D}{V_T}$ ratio indicates ventilation is in excess of perfusion. Emphysema, positive-pressure ventilation, pulmonary embolism, and hypotension are some causes of increased deadspace ventilation.

For patients receiving mechanical ventilation, $\frac{V_D}{V_T}$ ratio of up to 60% is considered acceptable. This value is consistent with a normal $\frac{V_D}{V_T}$ after the patient is weaned off mechanical ventilation.

## EQUATION

$$\frac{V_D}{V_T} = \frac{(P_aCO_2 - P_{\overline{E}}CO_2)}{P_aCO_2}$$

$\frac{V_D}{V_T}$ : Deadspace to tidal volume ratio in %

$P_aCO_2$ : Arterial carbon dioxide tension in mm Hg

$P_{\overline{E}}CO_2$ : Mixed expired carbon dioxide tension in mm Hg*

## NORMAL VALUE

20 to 40% in patients breathing spontaneously

40 to 60% in patients receiving mechanical ventilation

## EXAMPLE

Given: $P_aCO_2$ = 40 mm Hg

$P_{\overline{E}}CO_2$ = 30 mm Hg

Calculate the $\frac{V_D}{V_T}$ ratio.

$$\frac{V_D}{V_T} = \frac{(P_aCO_2 - P_{\overline{E}}CO_2)}{P_aCO_2}$$

$$= \frac{40 - 30}{40}$$

$$= \frac{10}{40}$$

$$= 0.25 \text{ or } 25\%$$

## EXERCISE

Given: $P_aCO_2$ = 30 mm Hg

$P_{\overline{E}}CO_2$ = 15 mm Hg

Calculate the $\frac{V_D}{V_T}$ ratio.

[Answer: $\frac{V_D}{V_T}$ = 0.50 or 50%]

**REFERENCES** Shapiro (1) (2)

*$P_{\bar{E}}CO_2$ is measured by analyzing the $PCO_2$ of a sample of expired gas collected on the exhalation port of the ventilator circuit or via a one-way valve for spontaneously breathing patients. A 5-L bag can be used for sample collection. To prevent contamination of the gas sample, sigh breaths should not be included in this sample and exhaled gas should be completely isolated from the patient circuit. The $P_aCO_2$ is measured by analyzing an arterial blood gas sample obtained while collecting the exhaled gas sample.*

## Self-Assessment Questions

18a. A mixed, expired gas sample for analysis of partial pressure of $CO_2$ is required for calculation of
(A) *I:E* ratio
(B) air entrainment ratio
(C) $V_D/V_T$ ratio
(D) cardiac index
(E) *a/A* ratio

18b. The deadspace to tidal volume ratio ($V_D/V_T$) requires measurements of:
I. Arterial $PCO_2$
II. Venous $PCO_2$
III. Mixed expired $PCO_2$
IV. Mixed expired $PO_2$
V. Arterial $PO_2$
(A) I, III only
(B) I, IV only
(C) II, III, IV only
(D) II, IV only
(E) II, III, V only

18c. For intubated patients who are being ventilated by a mechanical ventilator, it is acceptable to have a $V_D/V_T$ ratio of up to
(A) 20%
(B) 30%
(C) 40%
(D) 50%
(E) 60%

18d. Given: $P_aCO_2 = 35$ mm Hg, $P_{\bar{E}}CO_2 = 20$ mm Hg, $P_aO_2 = 80$ mm Hg, pH = 7.45. What is the $V_D/V_T$ ratio?
(A) 26%
(B) 31%

    (C) 35%

    (D) 43%

    (E) 75%

18e.  Given: $P_aCO_2 = 40$ mm Hg, $P\overline{E}CO_2 = 30$ mm Hg. Calculate the $V_D/V_T$ ratio.

    (A) 10%

    (B) 20%

    (C) 25%

    (D) 30%

    (E) 75%

18f.  A 55-year-old man was admitted to the hospital for shortness of breath. The following results were obtained: $P_aCO_2 = 50$ mm Hg, $P\overline{E}CO_2 = 30$ mm Hg. What is the calculated $V_D/V_T$ ratio?

    (A) 15%

    (B) 20%

    (C) 30%

    (D) 40%

    (E) 50%

18g.  A patient who is on a mechanical ventilator has the following measurements: $P_aCO_2 = 45$ mm Hg, $P\overline{E}CO_2 = 25$ mm Hg. What is the patient's deadspace to tidal volume ratio? Is it normal?

    (A) 44%; normal

    (B) 44%; abnormal

    (C) 55%; normal

    (D) 55%; abnormal

    (E) tidal volume required to calculate answer

CHAPTER

# *19*
# Density (*D*) of Gases

*NOTE*

The density of gas molecules is directly proportional to the molecular weights. In general, atoms and molecules having lower atomic numbers (smaller atomic weights) are lighter than those having higher atomic numbers. Atomic weight is also known as atomic mass.

## EQUATION

$$D = \frac{gmw \text{ (g)}}{22.4 \text{ (L)}}$$

$D$    : Density of gas in g / L

$gmw$  : Gram molecular weight in g*

## EXAMPLE 1

Calculate the density of carbon dioxide ($CO_2$).

$$D = \frac{gmw \text{ (g)}}{22.4 \text{ (L)}}$$

$$= \frac{\text{atomic weight of C} + (\text{atomic weight of O} \times 2)}{22.4}$$

$$= \frac{12 + (16 \times 2)}{22.4}$$

$$= \frac{12 + 32}{22.4}$$

$$= \frac{44}{22.4}$$

$$= 1.96 \text{ g/L}$$

## EXAMPLE 2

Calculate the density of air (21% $O_2$, 78% $N_2$, 1% Ar).

$$D = \frac{gmw \text{ (g)}}{22.4 \text{ (L)}}$$

$$= \frac{0.21 \times (\text{wt. of O} \times 2) + 0.78 \times (\text{wt. of N} \times 2) + 0.01 \times (\text{wt. of Ar})}{22.4}$$

$$= \frac{0.21 \times (16 \times 2) + 0.78 \times (14 \times 2) + 0.01 \times (40)}{22.4}$$

$$= \frac{0.21 \times 32 + 0.78 \times 28 + 0.01 \times 40}{22.4}$$

$$= \frac{6.72 + 21.84 + 0.4}{22.4}$$

$$= \frac{28.96}{22.4}$$

$$= 1.29 \text{ g/L}$$

*$gmw$ = *Atomic weight* × *Number of atoms per molecule.*

**EXERCISE 1**    Use the Periodic Chart of Elements in Appendix H and find the atomic weight and gram molecular weight (*gmw*) of oxygen ($O_2$).

[Answer: Atomic weight of O = 16 g; *gmw* of $O_2$ = 32 g]

**EXERCISE 2**    What is the density (*D*) of oxygen ($O_2$)?

[Answer: *D* = 1.429 g/L]

**EXERCISE 3**    Calculate the density of a gas mixture of 70% helium (He) and 30% oxygen ($O_2$).

[Answer: *D* = 0.554 g/L]

**REFERENCE**    Scanlan

**SEE**    *Appendix H, Periodic Chart of Elements.*

## Self-Assessment Questions

19a.  Calculate the density of nitrogen ($N_2$) if the atomic weight for nitrogen is 14.

    (A) 0.31 g/L

    (B) 0.63 g/L

    (C) 1.25 g/L

    (D) 2.5 g/L

    (E) 14 g/L

19b. Given: atomic weight of helium = 4 g. What is its gas density?

(A) 0.18 g/L

(B) 1.8 g/L

(C) 18 g/L

(D) 4 g/L

(E) 40 g/L

19c. Calculate the density of carbon dioxide ($CO_2$) given that the atomic weights for carbon and oxygen are 12 and 16, respectively.

(A) 1.48 g/L

(B) 1.61 g/L

(C) 1.75 g/L

(D) 1.96 g.L

(E) 2.14 g/L

19d. Calculate the density of a helium/oxygen mixture (80% He, 20% $O_2$). The atomic weights for helium and oxygen are 4 and 16, respectively.

(A) 0.43 g/L

(B) 0.52 g/L

(C) 0.68 g/L

(D) 0.79 g/L

(E) 0.81 g/L

19e. Which of the following gas element/molecules is the most dense? He, $N_2$, CO, $O_2$, $CO_2$. Calculate and report their densities. The molecular weights for He, $N_2$, CO, $O_2$, and $CO_2$ are 4, 28, 28, 32, and 44, respectively.

(A) He: 0.18 g/L

(B) $N_2$: 1.25 g/L

(C) CO: 1.25 g/L

(D) $O_2$: 1.43 g/L

(E) $CO_2$: 1.96 g/L

# *20*

# Dosage Calculation: Intravenous Solution Infusion Dosage

*NOTE*

The infusion dosage is usually in mg/min or μg/min. The dosage in 1 mL must first be converted to the proper unit (mg or μg) before using the equation (i.e., 1 g = 1000 mg; 1 mg = 1000 μg).

**EQUATION**

$$\text{Infusion dosage} = \frac{\text{Infusion rate} \times \text{Dosage in 1 mL}}{60 \text{ drops/mL}}$$

Infusion dosage : Infusion dosage of intravenous (IV) solution, in mg / min or μg / min

Infusion rate : Infusion rate of intravenous (IV) solution in drops / min

Dosage in 1 mL : Concentration of drug, in mg / mL or μg / mL

60 drops / mL : Represents 60 IV drops in 1 mL

**EXAMPLE 1**

A 10-mL ampule of bretylium tosylate containing 500 mg of drug is mixed in 250 mL of D5W. If an infusion rate of 30 drops / min is being administered to the patient, what is the infusion dosage per minute? Since 500 mg / 250 mL = 2 mg / mL, this is used below as dosage in 1 mL. (See Dosage Calculation: Percent (%) Solution for further discussion.)

$$\text{Infusion dosage} = \frac{\text{Infusion rate} \times \text{Dosage in 1 mL}}{60 \text{ drops/mL}}$$

$$= \frac{30 \text{ drops/min} \times 2 \text{ mg/mL}}{60 \text{ drops/mL}}$$

$$= \frac{60 \text{ mg/min}}{60}$$

$$= 1 \text{ mg/min}$$

**EXAMPLE 2**

1 mg of insoproterenol is mixed with 250 mL of D5W. If an infusion rate of 30 drops / min is being administered to the patient, what is the infusion dosage per minute?

Since 1 mg / 250 mL = 1000 μg / 250 mL = 4 μg / mL, this is used below as dosage in 1 mL. (See Dosage Calculation: Percent (%) Solution for further discussion.)

$$\text{Infusion dosage} = \frac{\text{Infusion rate} \times \text{Dosage in 1 mL}}{60 \text{ drops/mL}}$$

$$= \frac{30 \text{ drops/min} \times 4 \text{ } \mu g/mL}{60 \text{ drops/mL}}$$

$$= \frac{120 \text{ } \mu g/min}{60}$$

$$= 2 \text{ } \mu g/min$$

**EXERCISE 1**    A 2-mL vial of procainamide containing 1 g of drug is mixed in 250 mL of D5W. If an infusion rate of 30 drops/min is being administered to the patient, what is the infusion dosage in mg per minute?

[Answer: Infusion dosage = 2 mg/min]

**EXERCISE 2**    50 mg of Nipride are mixed with 250 mL of D5W. If an infusion rate of 3 drops/min is being given to the patient, what is the infusion dosage in μg per minute?

[Answer: Infusion dosage = 10 μg/min]

**REFERENCE**    Grauer

**SEE**    *Dosage Calculation: Percent (%) Solution; Dosage Calculation: Intravenous Solution Infusion Rate*

## Self-Assessment Questions

20a.  One gram of procainamide hydrochloride is mixed with 250 mL of D5W. If this mixture is given to a patient at an infusion rate of 15 drops/min, what is the infusion dosage in mg/min?

(A) 0.5 mg/min

(B) 1 mg/min

(C) 2 mg/min

(D) 2.5 mg/min

(E) 3 mg/min

20b.  50 mg (50,000 μg) of sodium nitroprusside are mixed with 250 mL of D5W. At an infusion rate of 6 drops/min, what is the infusion dosage in μg/min?

(A) 5 μg/min

(B) 10 μg/min

(C) 15 μg/min

(D) 20 μg/min

(E) 25 μg/min

20c.  A 250-mL D5W solution contains 1 ampule (200 mg) of dopamine hydrochloride. If the patient is receiving this IV solution at a rate of 18 drops/min, what is the infusion dosage in µg/min?

(A) 240 µg/min

(B) 260 µg/min

(C) 280 µg/min

(D) 300 µg/min

(E) 320 µg/min

20d.  50 mg of nitroglycerin are mixed with 250 mL of D5W, and the mixture is running at an infusion rate of 3 drops/min. What is the infusion dosage in µg/min?

(A) 5 µg/min

(B) 10 µg/min

(C) 15 µg/min

(D) 20 µg/min

(E) 25 µg/min

CHAPTER

# 21
# Dosage Calculation: Intravenous Solution Infusion Rate

## NOTES

It is essential to use the proper units (mg or µg) in the infusion dosage and dosage in 1 mL. To find dosage in 1 mL, 1 g is usually converted to 1000 mg and 1 mg to 1000 µg.

If the infusion dosage is related to a patient's *body weight* (i.e., n mg/kg/min or n µg/kg/min), multiply the n by the patient's body weight in kg and use the equation as shown in Example 2. For example, if the infusion dosage is 5 µg/kg/min, an 80-kg patient would require an infusion dosage of 400 µg/min (5 µg/kg/min × 80 kg).

## EQUATION

$$\text{Infusion rate} = \frac{60 \text{ drops/mL} \times \text{Infusion dosage}}{\text{dosage in 1 mL}}$$

| | | |
|---|---|---|
| Infusion rate | : | Infusion rate of intravenous (IV) solution in drops/min |
| 60 drops/mL | : | Represents 60 IV drops in 1 mL |
| Infusion dosage | : | Infusion dosage of intravenous (IV) solution, in mg/min or µg/min |
| Dosage in 1 mL | : | Concentration of drug, in mg/mL or µg/mL |

## EXAMPLE 1

1 g of lidocaine is mixed with 250 mL of D5W. If an infusion dosage of 2 mg/min is desired, what should be the infusion rate in drops/min? Since 1 g/250 mL = 1000 mg/250 mL = 4 mg/mL, this is used below as dosage in 1 mL.

$$\text{Infusion Rate} = \frac{60 \text{ drops/mL} \times \text{Infusion dosage}}{\text{Dosage in 1 mL}}$$

$$= \frac{60 \text{ drops/mL} \times 2 \text{ mg/min}}{4 \text{ mg/mL}}$$

$$= \frac{120 \text{ drops/mL} \times \text{mg/min}}{4 \text{ mg/mL}}$$

$$= 30 \text{ drops/min}$$

## EXAMPLE 2

200 mg (1 amp) of dopamine is mixed with 250 mL of D5W. If an infusion dosage of 5 µg/kg/min is desired, what should be the infusion rate in drops/min for a patient weighing 80 kg?

For an 80-kg patient, the infusion dosage of 5 µg/kg/min would become 400 µg/min (5 µg/kg/min × 80 kg).

Since 200 mg/250 mL = 200,000 μg/250 mL = 800 μg/mL, this is used below as dosage in 1 mL.

$$\text{Infusion Rate} = \frac{60 \text{ drops/mL} \times \text{Infusion dosage}}{\text{Dosage in 1 mL}}$$

$$= \frac{60 \text{ drops/mL} \times 400 \text{ μg/min}}{800 \text{ μg/mL}}$$

$$= \frac{24,000 \text{ drops/mL} \times \text{μg/min}}{800 \text{ μg/mL}}$$

$$= 30 \text{ drops/min}$$

## EXERCISE 1

Two 10-mL ampules of bretylium tosylate containing 500 mg of drug in each ampule is mixed with 250 mL of D5W, for a total amount of 1000 mg/250 mL. If an infusion dosage of 2 mg/min is desired, what should be the infusion rate in drops/min?

[Answer: Infusion rate = 30 drops/min]

## EXERCISE 2

1 mg of epinephrine is mixed with 250 mL of D5W. If an infusion dosage of 1 μg/min is desired, what should be the infusion rate in drops/min?

[Answer: Infusion rate = 15 drops/min]

## REFERENCE

Grauer

## SEE

*Dosage Calculation: Percent (%) Solution; Dosage Calculation: Intravenous Solution Infusion Dosage*

## Self-Assessment Questions

21a. One gram of lidocaine is mixed with 250 mL of D5W. At an infusion dosage of 1.6 mg/min intravenously, what should be the infusion rate in drops/min?

(A) 16 drops/min

(B) 18 drops/min

(C) 20 drops/min

(D) 22 drops / min

(E) 24 drops / min

21b. Two grams of bretylium tosylate are mixed with 500 mL of D5W for intravenous use. If an infusion dosage of 2 mg/min is desired, find the infusion rate in drops/min.

(A) 8 drops / min

(B) 24 drops / min

(C) 30 drops / min

(D) 40 drops / min

(E) 60 drops / min

21c. Find the infusion rate in drops/min when 1 mg of isoproterenol in 250 mL of D5W is used for an infusion dosage of 2 µg/min.

(A) 15 drops / min

(B) 20 drops / min

(C) 25 drops / min

(D) 30 drops / min

(E) 35 drops / min

21d. A 10-mL ampule of bretylium tosylate containing 500 mg of drug is mixed with 250 mL of D5W. If an infusion dosage of 1 mg/min is desired, what should be the infusion rate in drops/min?

(A) 25 drops / min

(B) 30 drops / min

(C) 35 drops / min

(D) 40 drops / min

(E) 45 drops / min

21e. A 250-mL D5W solution contains 1 mg of epinephrine. If an infusion dosage of 2 µg/min is needed, what should be the infusion rate in drops/min?

(A) 5 drops / min

(B) 15 drops / min

(C) 30 drops / min

(D) 40 drops / min

(E) 50 drops / min

CHAPTER

# 22
# Dosage Calculation: Percent (%) Solutions

*NOTES*

In Example 2, the volume calculated must be diluted with normal saline or other diluents before use. This applies to almost all respiratory care bronchodilator stock solutions.

Drug dosage calculation for unit dose is similar to that shown in the examples.

## EQUATION 1

Dosage = Volume used × Concentration of original solution

## EQUATION 2

$$\text{Volume} = \frac{\text{Dosage desired}}{\text{Concentration of original solution}}$$

## EXAMPLE 1

How many mg of isoproterenol are in 0.5 mL of a 1:100 (1%) drug solution?

SOLUTION A. [This calculation gives answer in g. It must be converted to mg.]

$$
\begin{aligned}
\text{Dosage} &= \text{Volume used} \times \text{Concentration of original solution} \\
&= 0.5 \times 1\% \\
&= 0.5 \times 0.01 \\
&= 0.005 \text{ g (or 5 mg)}
\end{aligned}
$$

SOLUTION B. The 1:100 or 1% solution can be rewritten as follows:

$$
\begin{aligned}
1\% &= \frac{1 \text{ g}}{100 \text{ mL}} \\
&= \frac{1000 \text{ mg}}{100 \text{ mL}} \\
&= 10 \text{ mg/mL}
\end{aligned}
$$

[This calculation gives answer in mg.]

$$
\begin{aligned}
\text{Dosage} &= \text{Volume used} \times \text{Concentration of original solution} \\
&= 0.5 \text{ mL} \times 1\% \\
&= 0.5 \text{ mL} \times 10 \text{ mg/mL} \\
&= 5 \text{ mg}
\end{aligned}
$$

## EXAMPLE 2

A stock bottle of isoproterenol has a concentration of 1:200. How much volume is needed if 2.5 mg of the active ingredient is desired?

$$
\begin{aligned}
\text{Volume} &= \frac{\text{Dosage desired}}{\text{Concentration of original solution}} \\
&= \frac{2.5 \text{ mg}}{1{:}200} \\
&= \frac{2.5 \text{ mg}}{(1 \text{ g}/200 \text{ mL})}
\end{aligned}
$$

$$= \frac{2.5 \text{ mg}}{(1000 \text{ mg}/200\text{mL}}$$

$$= \frac{2.5 \text{ mg}}{5 \text{ mg}/\text{mL}}$$

$$= 0.5 \text{ mL}$$

**EXERCISE 1**    How many mg of active ingredient are in 0.5 mL of a 0.5% albuterol sulfate solution?

[Answer: Dosage = 2.5 mg]

**EXERCISE 2**    What volume is needed from a 0.5% solution in order to obtain 5 mg of active ingredient?

[Answer: Volume = 1 mL]

**REFERENCE**    Rau

**SEE**    *Dosage Calculation: Unit Dose.*

## Self-Assessment Questions

22a.  A 1:1000 (0.1%) drug solution is the same as

(A) 0.01 mg/mL

(B)  0.1 mg/mL

(C)  1 mg/mL

(D) 10 mg/mL

(E)  100 mg/mL

22b.  How many mg of active ingredient are present in 0.5 mL of a 1:100 (1%) drug solution?

(A) 5 mg

(B)  10 mg

(C)  15 mg

(D) 20 mg

(E) 25 mg

22c.  How many mg of active ingredient are in 1 mL of a 1:200 drug solution?

(A) 1 mg

(B) 2 mg

(C) 5 mg

(D) 10 mg

(E) 50 mg

22d.  A stock bottle of albuterol sulfate has a concentration of 1:200 (0.5%). How much volume should be drawn from the bottle if 20 mg of the active ingredient are needed?

(A) 0.5 mL

(B) 1 mL

(C) 2 mL

(D) 3 mL

(E) 4 mL

22e.  How many mg of active ingredient are present in 8 mL of a 0.5% albuterol sulfate solution?

(A) 10 mg

(B) 20 mg

(C) 30 mg

(D) 40 mg

(E) 50 mg

22f.  What volume is needed from a 0.5% drug solution in order to obtain 5 mg of active ingredient?

(A) 0.25 mL

(B) 0.5 mL

(C) 1 mL

(D) 1.5 mL

(E) 2 mL

22g.  A stock bottle of albuterol sulfate has a concentration of 1:200 (0.5%). How many mg of active ingredient are present in a HEART (High-output extended aerosol respiratory therapy) treatment if 4 mL of this bronchodilator are used?

(A) 5 mg

(B) 10 mg

(C) 15 mg

(D) 20 mg

(E) 40 mg

22h.  How much of a 1% solution of isoetharine is needed in order to obtain 5 mg of active ingredient?

(A) 0.25 mL

(B) 0.5 mL

(C) 1 mL

(D) 1.5 mL

(E) 2 mL

22i. The physician orders 0.25 mL of isoetharine to be diluted in NaCl for a 1-year-old child. If a 1% isoetharine solution is used to prepare this mixture, how much active ingredient is used?

(A) 0.25 mg

(B) 0.5 mg

(C) 1 mg

(D) 1.5 mg

(E) 2.5 mg

22j. A stock bottle of racemic epinephrine has a concentration of 2.25%. How much of this solution is needed in order to obtain 10 mg of active ingredient?

(A) 0.22 mL

(B) 0.33 mL

(C) 0.44 mL

(D) 0.5 mL

(E) 0.75 mL

22k. The physician orders 0.15 mL of racemic epinephrine with normal saline for a child admitted for croup. If the racemic epinephrine solution has a concentration of 2.25%, about how much active ingredient is ordered?

(A) 0.34 mg

(B) 1.57 mg

(C) 2.25 mg

(D) 3.38 mg

(E) 4.54 mg

22l. A 10-mL bottle of 5% metaproterenol is used to prepare a dosage of 20 mg of this bronchodilator. How much of this solution should be used?

(A) 0.2 mL

(B) 0.3 mL

(C) 0.4 mL

(D) 0.5 mL

(E) 0.6 mL

22m. A stock bottle of metaproterenol sulfate contains a 5% solution. If 0.3 mL of this drug is used, it is the same as

(A) 1.5 mg

(B) 2.5 mg

(C) 5 mg

(D) 10 mg

(E) 15 mg

CHAPTER

# 23
# Dosage Calculation: Unit Dose

**EQUATION 1**  Dosage = Volume used × Concentration of unit dose

**EQUATION 2**  $Volume = \dfrac{Dosage\ desired}{Concentration\ of\ unit\ dose}$

**EXAMPLE 1**  A unit dose of isoetharine contains 2.5 mL of a 0.2% solution. How many mg of active ingredient are in this unit dose?

SOLUTION A. [This calculation gives answer in g. It must be converted to mg.]

Dosage = Volume used × Concentration of unit dose

= 2.5 mL × 0.2%

= 2.5 mL × 0.002 g / mL

= 0.005 g (or 5 mg)

SOLUTION B. The 0.2% solution can be rewritten as follows:

$0.2\% = \dfrac{0.2\ g}{100\ mL}$

$= \dfrac{200\ mg}{100\ mg}$

$= 2\ mg/mL$

[This calculation gives answer in mg.]

Dosage = Volume used × Concentration of unit dose

= 2.5 mL × 0.2%

= 2.5 mL × 2 mg / mL

= 5 mg

**EXAMPLE 2**  A unit dose of albuterol sulfate contains 3.0 mL of a 0.83 mg / mL solution. How many mg of active ingredient are in this unit dose?

Dosage = Volume used × Concentration of unit dose

= 3.0 mL × 0.83 mg / mL

= 2.49 or 2.5 mg

## EXAMPLE 3

A unit dose of albuterol sulfate contains 3.0 mL of a 0.83 mg/mL solution. How much volume is needed if 1.5 mg of the active ingredient is desired?

$$\text{Volume} = \frac{\text{Dosage desired}}{\text{Concentration of unit dose}}$$

$$= \frac{1.5 \text{ mg}}{0.83 \text{ mg/mL}}$$

$$= 1.8 \text{ mL}$$

## EXERCISE 1

A metaproterenol sulfate unit dose contains 2.5 mL of a 0.6% concentration. How many mg of active ingredient are in this unit dose? How much active ingredient is in half of a unit dose?

[Answer: Dosage = 15 mg; $\frac{1}{2}$ unit dose = 7.5 mg]

## EXERCISE 2

A unit dose of albuterol sulfate has 3.0 mL of a 0.83 mg/mL concentration. What is the total amount of active ingredient in this unit dose?

[Answer: Dosage in 3.0 mL = 2.49 or 2.5 mg]

## EXERCISE 3

A 3.0 mL unit dose of albuterol sulfate has a concentration of 0.83 mg/mL. How much of this unit dose should be used if 1.66 mg of active ingredient are needed?

[Answer: Volume of unit dose needed = 2 mL]

## REFERENCE

Rau

# Self-Assessment Questions

23a. A unit dose of bronchodilator contains 5.0 mL of a 0.5 mg/mL solution. How much active ingredient is in this unit dose?

(A) 0.5 mg

(B) 1.0 mg

(C) 2.5 mg

(D) 5.0 mg

(E) 10.0 mg

23b. A unit dose of isoetharine contains 2.5 mL of a 0.2% solution. How many mg of active ingredient are present in this unit dose?

(A) 1.25 mg

(B) 2.5 mg

(C) 5 mg

(D) 10 mg

(E) 25 mg

23c. A unit dose of albuterol sulfate contains 3.0 mL of a 0.083% solution. How many mg of active ingredient are present in this unit dose?

(A) 1.5 mg

(B) 2.5 mg

(C) 5 mg

(D) 10 mg

(E) 25 mg

23d. A unit dose of albuterol sulfate contains 3.0 mL of a 0.083% solution. How many unit doses are needed in order to obtain 20 mg of the active ingredient?

(A) 4 unit doses

(B) 6 unit doses

(C) 8 unit doses

(D) 10 unit doses

(E) 12 unit doses

23e. A metaproterenol sulfate unit dose contains 2.5 mL of a 0.6% solution. How many mg of active ingredient are present in this unit dose?

(A) 0.6 mg

(B) 2.5 mg

(C) 5 mg

(D) 10 mg

(E) 15 mg

23f. A unit dose of albuterol sulfate contains 3.0 mL of a 0.083% solution. If eight unit doses are used in a HEART (High-output extended aerosol respiratory therapy) treatment, what is the total amount of active ingredient in the nebulizer?

(A) 2.5 mg

(B) 5 mg

(C) 10 mg

(D) 20 mg

(E) 40 mg

23g. A unit dose of albuterol sulfate contains 3.0 mL of a 0.083% solution. If 2 unit doses are used, how many mg of active ingredient are used?

(A) 2.75 mg

(B) 5 mg

(C) 7.5 mg

(D) 12.5 mg

(E) 15 mg

23h. Each ampule of Brethine (terbutaline sulfate) contains 1 mL of a 0.1% solution. What is the total dosage if two ampules (2 mL) are used?

(A) 1 mg

(B) 2 mg

(C) 3 mg

(D) 4 mg

(E) 5 mg

23i. The physician orders 0.5 mL of a unit dose of Brethine (terbutaline sulfate) with saline for a pediatric patient. If the 1 mL unit dose ampule comes in a 0.1% solution, how many mg of this drug are used?

(A) 0.01 mg

(B) 0.1 mg

(C) 0.5 mg

(D) 1.0 mg

(E) 2 mg

23j. An atropine sulfate unit dose contains 1 mL of a 0.1% solution. How many mg of active ingredient are in $\frac{3}{4}$ of a unit dose?

(A) 0.01 mg

(B) 0.1 mg

(C) 0.5 mg

(D) 0.75 mg

(E) 1 mg

23k. The physician orders two unit doses of atropine sulfate. If each unit dose contains 1 mg/mL of active ingredient, how many mg of atropine sulfate are ordered?

(A) 0.1 mg

(B) 0.2 mg

(C) 1 mg

(D) 2 mg

(E) 20 mg

23l. A unit dose of liquid Intal (cromolyn sodium) contains 20 mg/2 mL. How much active ingredient is in 1 mL of this solution?

(A) 1 mg

(B) 5 mg

(C) 10 mg

(D) 20 mg

(E) 40 mg

23m. What is the total amount of cromolyn sodium in two unit doses if each 2-mL unit dose contains 20 mg?

(A) 1 mg

(B) 5 mg

(C) 10 mg

(D) 20 mg

(E) 40 mg

# 24
# Dosage Estimation for Children: Young's Rule

**EQUATION**

$$\text{Child's dose} = \left[\frac{\text{Age}}{(\text{Age} + 12)}\right] \times \text{Adult dose}$$

Child's dose : Estimated child's drug dosage
Age : Age of child in years
Adult dose : Normal adult drug dosage

**EXAMPLE**

What should be the dosage for an 8-year-old if the adult dose is 50 mg?

$$\text{Child's dose} = \left[\frac{\text{Age}}{(\text{Age} + 12)}\right] \times \text{Adult dose}$$
$$= \left[\frac{8}{(8 + 12)}\right] \times 50 \text{ mg}$$
$$= \left[\frac{8}{20}\right] \times 50 \text{ mg}$$
$$= 0.4 \times 50 \text{ mg}$$
$$= 20 \text{ mg}$$

**EXERCISE**

If the adult dose is 30 mg, what is the calculated pediatric dose for a 6-year-old patient?

[Answer: Dosage = 10 mg]

**REFERENCE**

Hegstad

## Self-Assessment Questions

24a.  If the child's age is known and is within the range of 1 to 12 years, the drug dosage for this child can be estimated by using

(A) Old's rule

(B) Young's rule

(C) Clark's rule

(D) Fried's rule

(E) Robert's rule

24b.  If the drug dosage for an adult is 15 mg, what is the pediatric dosage for a 6-year-old patient using Young's rule for dosage calculation?

(A) 1 mg

(B) 2 mg

(C) 5 mg

(D) 10 mg

(E) 15 mg

24c.  Using Young's rule of dosage calculation for children, what should be the dosage for a 5-year-old child if the adult dose of a medication is 10 mg?

(A) 1.88 or 1.9 mg

(B) 2.45 or 2.5 mg

(C) 2.94 or 2.9 mg

(D) 3.07 or 3.1 mg

(E) 4.78 or 4.8 mg

24d.  If the adult dosage of a medication is 25 mg, what should be the dosage for a 10-year-old child based on Young's rule of dosage calculation for children?

(A) 11.36 or 11 mg

(B) 12.41 or 12 mg

(C) 13.09 or 13 mg

(D) 14.44 or 14 mg

(E) 14.87 or 15 mg

CHAPTER

# 25
# Dosage Estimation for Infants and Children: Clark's Rule

*NOTES*

Clark's rule of dosage calculation requires the infant's or child's *weight*. Clark's rule can be used in infants and children. It provides a more reasonable estimate of drug dosage than Young's rule when the patient's body weight is not in proportion to age.

Since an effective drug dosage varies greatly among individuals and conditions, the calculated dosage must be carefully evaluated before drug administration.

**EQUATION**

$$\text{Infant's or child's dose} = \left(\frac{\text{Weight in lb}}{150}\right) \times \text{Adult dose}$$

| | | |
|---|---|---|
| Infant's or child's dose | : | Estimated infant's or child's dosage |
| Weight in lb | : | Weight of infant or child in pounds |
| Adult dose | : | Normal adult drug dosage |
| 150 | : | A constant number |

**EXAMPLE**

What should be the dosage for a 50-lb child if the adult dose is 30 mg?

$$\text{Infant's or child's dose} = \left(\frac{\text{Weight in lb}}{150}\right) \times \text{Adult dose}$$

$$= \left(\frac{50}{150}\right) \times 30 \text{ mg}$$

$$= \frac{1}{3} \times 30 \text{ mg}$$

$$= 10 \text{ mg}$$

**EXERCISE**

If the adult dose is 50 mg, what is the calculated dosage for a 3-lb infant?

[Answer: Dosage = 1 mg]

**REFERENCE**

Hegstad

# Self-Assessment Questions

25a. With Clark's rule of dosage calculation for infants and children, what should be the dosage for a 6-lb infant if the adult dose is 30 mg?

(A) 1.2 mg

(B) 1.8 mg

(C) 2.4 mg

(D) 3.0 mg

(E) 3.6 mg

25b. Use Clark's rule of dosage calculation for infants and children to calculate the dosage for a 50-lb child. The normal adult dose is 30 mg.

(A) 2 mg

(B) 4 mg

(C) 6 mg

(D) 8 mg

(E) 10 mg

25c. If the weight of an infant or child is known, the drug dosage for this infant or child can be estimated by using

(A) Young's rule

(B) Rules of sevens

(C) Clark's rule

(D) Pickwick's rule

(E) Fried's rule

CHAPTER

# 26
# Dosage Estimation for Infants and Children: Fried's Rule

Fried's rule of dosage calculation requires the infant's or child's *age in months*. Fried's rule can be used for infants and children up to 2 years of age.

If the body weight of the infant or child is not in proportion to age, Clark's rule for dosage calculation should be used.

Since an effective drug dosage varies greatly among individuals and conditions, the calculated dosage must be carefully evaluated before drug administration.

## EQUATION

$$\text{Infant's or child's dose} = \left( \frac{\text{Age in months}}{150} \right) \times \text{Adult dose}$$

| | | |
|---|---|---|
| Infant's or child's dose | : | Estimated infant's or child's dosage |
| Age in months | : | Age of infant or child in months, up to 24 months |
| Adult dose | : | Normal adult drug dosage |
| 150 | : | A constant number |

## EXAMPLE

What should be the dosage for a 15-month-old child if the adult dose is 30 mg?

$$\text{Infant's or child's dose} = \left( \frac{\text{Age in months}}{150} \right) \times \text{Audlt dose}$$

$$= \left( \frac{15}{150} \right) \times 30 \text{ mg}$$

$$= \frac{1}{10} \times 30 \text{ mg}$$

$$= 3 \text{ mg}$$

## EXERCISE

If the adult dose is 50 mg, what is the calculated dosage for a 2-year-old child?

[Answer: Dosage = 8 mg]

## REFERENCE

Hegstad

## SEE

*Dosage Estimation for Infants and Children: Clark's Rule.*

## Self-Assessment Questions

26a. Based on Fried's rule, what should be the dosage for a 2-year-old toddler if the adult dose is 35 mg?

(A) 3.9 mg

(B) 4.7 mg

(C) 5.1 mg

(D) 5.6 mg

(E) 6.8 mg

26b. Use Fried's rule to estimate the dosage for a 15-month-old infant if the adult dose is 30 mg.

(A) 1 mg

(B) 2 mg

(C) 3 mg

(D) 4 mg

(E) 5 mg

26c. According to Fried's rule, the estimated dosage for a 5-month-old infant at an adult dose of 30 mg is

(A) 1 mg

(B) 2 mg

(C) 3 mg

(D) 4 mg

(E) 5 mg

26d. For infants and children up to 2 years old, the age in months may be used to estimate the drug dosage by using

(A) Young's rule

(B) Starling's rule

(C) Clark's rule

(D) DuBois's rule

(E) Fried's rule

# CHAPTER

# 27
# Elastance (*E*)

The elastance equation is modified from Hooke's law of elastic behavior, and it is expressed as the reciprocal of compliance.

When the lungs are stiff (non-compliant) the elastance (*E*) of the lungs is high and a high inflating pressure ($\Delta P$) is required to deliver a set volume ($\Delta V$). On the other hand, when the lungs are compliant, as in emphysema, the elastance of the lungs is low. In this situation, a high inflating pressure may be detrimental to the patient (e.g., barotrauma).

Compliance (*C*) is more commonly used to describe the elastic properties of the lungs.

## EQUATION

$$E = \frac{\Delta P}{\Delta V}$$

$E$    :   Elastance in cm $H_2O$ / L

$\Delta P$   :   Pressure change in cm $H_2O$

$\Delta V$   :   Volume change in mL or L

## NORMAL VALUE

5 to 10 cm $H_2O$/L

If the patient is intubated, use serial measurements to establish trend.

## EXAMPLE

Given: $\Delta P$ = 5 cm $H_2O$

$\Delta V$ = 0.8 L

Calculate the elastance.

$$E = \frac{\Delta P}{\Delta V}$$

$$= \frac{5}{0.8}$$

$$= 6.25 \text{ cm } H_2O/\text{ L}$$

## EXERCISE

Given: $\Delta P$ =   3 cm $H_2O$

$\Delta V$      =   0.6 L

Calculate the elastance.

[Answer: $E$ = 5 cm $H_2O$/L]

## REFERENCE

Burton

**SEE**           *Compliance: Dynamic ($C_{dyn}$); Compliance: Static ($C_{st}$)*

## Self-Assessment Questions

27a. Calculate the elastance if the change in pressure ($\Delta P$) is 10 cm $H_2O$ and change in volume ($\Delta V$) is 0.5 L. Is it normal?

(A) 20 cm $H_2O$/L; abnormal

(B) 10 cm $H_2O$/L; normal

(C) 5 cm $H_2O$/L; normal

(D) 10 L/cm $H_2O$; abnormal

(E) 20 L/cm $H_2O$; abnormal

27b. Calculate the elastance if the change in pressure ($\Delta P$) is 5 cm $H_2O$ and change in volume ($\Delta V$) is 0.7 L. Is it normal?

(A) 3.5 cm $H_2O$/L; abnormal

(B) 5 cm $H_2O$/L; normal

(C) 7.1 cm $H_2O$/L; normal

(D) 8.9 L/cm $H_2O$; abnormal

(E) 20 L/cm $H_2O$; abnormal

CHAPTER

# 28
# Endotracheal Tube Size for Children

This equation is used to esti-mate the size of an endotra-cheal (ET) tube for a child over 1 year old. The calcu-lated size should be adjusted up or down by 0.5 mm for dif-ferent body sizes. In an emer-gency situation, an ET tube may be selected by matching one with the diameter of a child's little finger.

Since ET tubes come in 0.5-mm increments, the esti-mated *ID* size should be rounded to the nearest whole or half size.

For neonates, the endotra-cheal tube size is not calcu-lated. Rather, Table 4 shows the general rule for selecting an appropriate endotracheal tube for a neonate.

## EQUATION 1

$$ID = \frac{Age + 16}{4}$$

or

## EQUATION 2

$$ID = \frac{Height}{20}$$

| | |
|---|---|
| *ID* | : Internal diameter of endotracheal tube in mm |
| Age | : Age of child over 1 year old, in years |
| Height | : Height of child in cm |

## EXAMPLE 1

What is the estimated size of an endotracheal tube for a 3-year-old child?

$$ID = \frac{Age + 16}{4}$$

$$= \frac{3 + 16}{4}$$

$$= \frac{19}{4}$$

$$= 4.75 \text{ or } 5.0 \text{ mm}$$

## EXAMPLE 2

What is the estimated size of an endotracheal tube for a child who is 4 ft* (about 120 cm) tall?

$$ID = \frac{Height}{20}$$

$$= \frac{120}{20}$$

$$l = 6.0 \text{ mm}$$

*1 ft = 12 in. and 1 in. = 2.54 cm.

**EXERCISE 1**    Calculate the estimated ET tube size for a 6-year-old child.

[Answer: *ID* = 5.5 mm]

**EXERCISE 2**    Calculate the estimated ET tube size for a child 3 ft (90 cm) tall.

[Answer: *ID* = 4.5 mm]

**TABLE 4. Endotracheal Tube Size for Neonates**

| BODY WEIGHT | ET SIZE (*ID mm*) |
|---|---|
| < 1,000 g | 2.5 |
| 1,000 to 2,000 g | 3.0 |
| 2,000 to 3,000 g | 3.5 |
| > 3,000 g | 4.0 |

**REFERENCES**    Koff; Whitaker

## Self-Assessment Questions

28a.  Calculate the estimated size of an endotracheal tube for a 2-year-old child.

   (A)  3.0 mm

   (B)  3.5 mm

   (C)  4.0 mm

   (D)  4.5 mm

   (E)  5.0 mm

28b.  For an 8-year-old child, the calculated size of an endotracheal tube is about

   (A)  4.5 mm

   (B)  5.0 mm

   (C)  5.5 mm

   (D)  6.0 mm

   (E)  6.5 mm

28c.  Calculate the estimated size of an endotracheal tube for a child who is 3 ft 6 in. (about 106 cm) tall.

(A) 3.5 mm

(B) 4.0 mm

(C) 4.5 mm

(D) 5.0 mm

(E) 6.0 mm

28d.  What should be the size of an endotracheal tube for a child who is 2 ft 6 in. (about 76 cm) tall?

(A) 3.5 mm

(B) 4.0 mm

(C) 4.5 mm

(D) 5.0 mm

(E) 5.5 mm

# CHAPTER

# *29*

# Fick's Law of Diffusion

## NOTES

Gas diffusion rate is directly related to the cross-sectional area of the lung membrane, the diffusion coefficient of gas, and the pressure gradient. It is inversely related to the thickness across the lung membrane.

## EQUATION

$$\text{Diffusion} = \frac{A \times D \times \Delta P}{T}$$

Diffusion : Gas diffusion rate

$A$ : Cross-sectional area of lung membrane

*Cross-sectional area of lung membrane (A)* In emphysema, some lung tissues are destroyed and the overall cross-sectional area of the lungs is diminished. The diffusion rate for these patients measured in the pulmonary function laboratory is therefore usually low.

$D$ : Diffusion coefficient of a gas

*Diffusion coefficient of a gas (D)* Carbon monoxide (CO) is used in gas diffusion studies due to its high diffusion rate and its ability to combine readily with hemoglobin (250 times greater than that of oxygen). CO is known as a diffusion-limited gas because its diffusion rate in the lungs is limited only by conditions in which the cross-sectional area of the lung membrane or the thickness across the lung membrane is affected.

$\Delta P$ : Pressure gradient of a gas

*Pressure gradient of a gas ($\Delta P$)* Pressure gradient of a gas is the fundamental principle of gas diffusion and exchange. Gas diffusion in the lungs and in the tissues follows the basic rule of pressure gradient: From an area of high pressure to an area of low pressure. In the pulmonary circulation, oxygen diffuses from alveoli ($P_AO_2 > 100$ mm Hg) to pulmonary capillaries ($P_{\bar{v}}O_2 = 40$ mm Hg), and carbon dioxide diffuses from pulmonary capillaries ($P_{\bar{v}}CO_2 = 46$ mm Hg) to alveoli ($P_ACO_2 = 40$ mm Hg). Oxygen therapy relies on this principle by increasing the pressure gradient of oxygen between the alveoli and pulmonary capillaries. A higher oxygen diffusion gradient facilitates oxygen diffusion into the pulmonary capillaries, and oxygenation of the mixed venous blood is therefore enhanced.

$T$ : Thickness across lung membrane

*Thickness across lung membrane (T)* Gas diffusion is hindered when the thickness across the lung membrane is increased. Pulmonary or interstitial edema, consolidation, and pulmonary fibrosis are some clinical conditions accompanied by an increase in thickness across the lung membrane. Oxygen therapy is not very effective in these conditions because oxygen, having a low diffusion coefficient, cannot diffuse across these lung units very well.

**REFERENCES** Des Jardins; Scanlan

**SEE** *Graham's Law of Diffusion Coefficient.*

## Self-Assessment Questions

29a. The diffusion rate of oxygen across the alveolar-capillary membrane is directly related to all of the following factors *except*
(A) diffusion coefficient of oxygen

(B) cross-sectional area of lung membrane

(C) alveolar-capillary pressure gradient of oxygen

(D) thickness across lung membrane

(E) inspired oxygen concentration ($F_IO_2$)

29b. In emphysema patients, the diffusion rate of gases across the alveolar-capillary membrane is lower than normal primarily due to
(A) airway obstruction

(B) increased diffusion coefficient of oxygen

(C) hypoventilation

(D) acidosis

(E) reduction of cross-sectional area of lung membrane

29c. In a pulmonary function laboratory, the gas diffusion rate is usually determined by using _____ because of its _____ diffusion coefficient.
(A) carbon monoxide; high

(B) carbon monoxide; low

(C) carbon dioxide; high

(D) oxygen; high

(E) oxygen; low

29d. Under normal conditions, the pressure gradient of oxygen between the arterial and mixed venous blood is about _____ mm Hg, considerably _____ than that of carbon dioxide.
(A) 60; lower

(B) 60; higher

(C) 40; lower

(D) 40; higher

(E) 20; lower

29e. A patient who is diagnosed with pneumonia has retained a large amount of secretions. This condition hinders gas diffusion and causes hypoxemia due to an increase of the

(A) diffusion coefficient of oxygen

(B) cross-sectional area of lung membrane

(C) pressure gradient of oxygen

(D) thickness across lung membrane

(E) alveolar $PO_2$

# CHAPTER

# *30*

# $F_IO_2$ from Two Gas Sources

*NOTE*

This equation is useful when a special oxygen setup involves two gas sources and an oxygen analyzer is not readily available.

## EQUATION

$$F_IO_2 = \frac{(\text{1st } F_IO_2 \times \text{1st flow}) + (\text{2nd } F_IO_2 \times \text{2nd flow})}{\text{Total flow}}$$

$F_IO_2$ : Inspired oxygen concentration in %

1st $F_IO_2$ : Oxygen concentration of 1st gas source in %

1st flow : Flow rate of 1st gas source in L/min

2nd $F_IO_2$ : Oxygen concentration of 2nd gas source in %

2nd flow : Flow rate of 2nd gas source in L/min

## EXAMPLE 1

What is the final $F_IO_2$ if 8 L/min of air is mixed with 2 L/min of oxygen?

$$F_IO_2 = \frac{(\text{1st } F_IO_2 \times \text{1st flow}) + (\text{2nd } F_IO_2 \times \text{2nd flow})}{\text{Total flow}}$$

$$= \frac{(0.21 \times 8) + (1.00 \times 2)}{(8 + 2)}$$

$$= \frac{1.68 + 2}{10}$$

$$= \frac{3.68}{10}$$

$$= 0.368 \text{ or } 37\%$$

## EXAMPLE 2

If the oxygen:air entrainment ratio is 1:10, what is the $F_IO_2$?

$$F_IO_2 = \frac{(\text{1st } F_IO_2 \times \text{1st flow}) + (\text{2nd } F_IO_2 \times \text{2nd flow})}{\text{Total flow}}$$

$$= \frac{(1.00 \times 1) + (0.21 \times 10)}{(1 + 10)}$$

$$= \frac{1 + 2.1}{11}$$

$$= \frac{3.1}{11}$$

$$= 0.28 \text{ or } 28\%$$

**EXAMPLE 2**

Calculate the $F_I O_2$ when 6 L/min of 40% oxygen is mixed with 2 L/min of air.

$$F_I O_2 = \frac{(\text{1st } F_I O_2 \times \text{1st flow}) + (\text{2nd } F_I O_2 \times \text{2nd flow})}{\text{Total flow}}$$

$$= \frac{(0.40 \times 6) + (0.21 \times 2)}{(6 + 2)}$$

$$= \frac{2.4 + 0.42}{8}$$

$$= \frac{2.82}{8}$$

$$= 0.353 \text{ or } 35\%$$

**EXERCISE 1**

If 3 L/min of 28% oxygen is mixed with 6 L/min of air, what is the final $F_I O_2$?

[Answer: $F_I O_2 = 0.233$ or 23%]

**EXERCISE 2**

Calculate the $F_I O_2$ when 6 L/min of 60% oxygen is mixed with 4 L/min of air.

[Answer: $F_I O_2 = 0.444$ or 44%]

**REFERENCE**

Barnes

**SEE**

*Oxygen:Air ($O_2$:Air) Entrainment Ratio.*

## Self-Assessment Questions

30a. What is the final oxygen concentration if 5 L/min of air is mixed with 5 L/min of oxygen?

(A) 20%

(B) 30%

(C) 40%

(D) 50%

(E) 60%

30b. What is the approximate $F_IO_2$ when 6 L/min of air is mixed with 2 L/min of oxygen?

(A) 30%

(B) 35%

(C) 40%

(D) 45%

(E) 50%

30c. Calculate the $F_IO_2$ when 1 L/min of oxygen is mixed with 4 L/min of air.

(A) 32%

(B) 37%

(C) 41%

(D) 46%

(E) 58%

30d. If the oxygen:air entrainment ratio is 1:10, what is the $F_IO_2$?

(A) 22%

(B) 24%

(C) 26%

(D) 28%

(E) 31%

30e. Which of the following oxygen:air entrainment ratios provides an $F_IO_2$ of 60%?

(A) 1 : 0.5

(B) 1 : 1

(C) 1 : 1.5

(D) 1 : 2

(E) 1 : 2.5

# CHAPTER

# *31*
# $F_IO_2$ Needed for a Desired $P_aO_2$

## NOTES

This two-step calculation is used to estimate the $F_IO_2$ needed to obtain a desired $P_aO_2$.

This calculation is useful to estimate the $F_IO_2$ needed in hypoxemia caused by hypoventilation or venous admixture (*V/Q* mismatch). In severe intrapulmonary shunts, this method is less dependable; positive end-expiratory pressure (PEEP) or continuous positive airway pressure (*CPAP*) may be needed for corrections of intrapulmonary shunting.

$$F_IO_2 = \frac{P_AO_2 \text{ needed} + (P_aCO_2 \times 1.25)}{P_B - 47}$$

## EQUATION 1

$$P_AO_2 \text{ needed} = \frac{P_aO_2 \text{ desired}}{a/A \text{ ratio}*}$$

## EQUATION 2

$$F_IO_2 = \frac{P_AO_2 \text{ needed} + 50}{713}$$

$P_AO_2$ needed : Alveolar oxygen tension needed for a desired $P_aO_2$.

$P_aO_2$ desired : Arterial oxygen tension desired

*a/A* ratio : Arterial/alveolar oxygen tension ratio in %

$F_IO_2$ : Inspired oxygen concentration needed to get a desired $P_aO_2$

## EXAMPLE

Given: *a/A* ratio = 0.55. What should be the $F_IO_2$ if a $P_aO_2$ of 100 mm Hg is desired?

$$(1)\ P_AO_2 \text{ needed} = \frac{P_aO_2 \text{ desired}}{a/A \text{ ratio}}$$

$$= \frac{100}{0.55}$$

$$= 182 \text{ mm hg}$$

$$(2)\ F_IO_2 \text{ needed} = \frac{P_AO_2 \text{ needed} + 50}{713}$$

$$= \frac{182 + 50}{713}$$

$$= \frac{232}{713}$$

$$= 0.325 \text{ or } 33\%$$

## EXERCISE

Given: $a/A$ ratio = 0.30. What should be the $F_IO_2$ if a $P_aO_2$ of 80 mm Hg is desired?

[Answer: $F_IO_2 = 0.44$ or 44%]

## REFERENCES

Burton; Krider

*See Arterial/Alveolar Oxygen Tension (a/A) Ratio.*
*For unusual $P_aCO_2$ or barometric pressure ($P_B$), use $F_IO_2$ equation*
*under Notes.*

## Self-Assessment Questions

31a.  Given: $a/A$ ratio = 0.35. What should be the $F_IO_2$ if a $P_aO_2$ of 100 mm Hg is desired?

(A) 27%

(B) 38%

(C) 47%

(D) 55%

(E) 66%

31b.  Given: $a/A$ ratio = 0.35. What should be the $F_IO_2$ if a $P_aO_2$ of 50 mm Hg is desired?

(A) 27%

(B) 38%

(C) 47%

(D) 55%

(E) 66%

31c.  The $a/A$ ratio is a patient is 0.80. If a $P_aO_2$ of 80 mm Hg is desired. what should be the $F_IO_2$? Is oxygen therapy necessary?

(A) 21%; not necessary

(B) 24%; necessary

(C) 28%; necessary

(D) 32%; necessary

(E) 35%; necessary

# *32*
# *$F_IO_2$ Needed for a Desired $P_aO_2$ (COPD patients)*

## NOTE

This calculation is used to estimate the $F_IO_2$ needed to obtain a low-range (50 to 60 mm Hg) $P_aO_2$—a value most suitable for COPD patients with uncomplicated acute exacerbation. To use this equation, a recent room air $P_aO_2$ must be known.

In this equation, the unit for $P_aO_2$ (mm Hg) is not used and is replaced by percent (%).

## EQUATION

$$F_IO_2 = 21\% + \left[\frac{(P_aO_2 \text{ desired} - \text{Room air } P_aO_2)}{3}\right]\%$$

$F_IO_2$ : Inspired oxygen concentration needed to get a desired $P_aO_2$, in %

$P_aO_2$ desired : Arterial oxygen tension desired

Room air $P_aO_2$ : Arterial oxygen tension on 21% oxygen

## EXAMPLE

Given: Room air $P_aO_2 = 45$ mm Hg. What should be the $F_IO_2$ if a $P_aO_2$ of 60 mm Hg is desired?

$$F_IO_2 = 21\% + \left[\frac{(P_aO_2 \text{ desired} - \text{Room air } P_aO_2)}{3}\right]\%$$

$$= 21\% + \left[\frac{(60 - 45)}{3}\right]\%$$

$$= 21\% + \left[\frac{15}{3}\right]\%$$

$$= 21\% + 5\%$$

$$= 26\%$$

## EXERCISE

Given: Room air $P_aO_2 = 35$ mm Hg. Estimate the $F_IO_2$ needed for a $P_aO_2$ of 55 mm Hg.

[Answer: $F_IO_2 = 28\%$]

## REFERENCE

Malley

## *Self-Assessment Questions*

32a.  The room-air $P_aO_2$ of a COPD patient is 40 mm Hg. What should be the $F_IO_2$ if a $P_aO_2$ of 60 mm Hg is desired?

(A) 22%

(B) 24%

(C) 26%

(D) 28%

(E) 31%

32b.  The $P_aO_2$ of a COPD patient is 40 mm Hg at an $F_IO_2$ of 21%. If a $P_aO_2$ of 55 mm Hg is desired, calculate the $F_IO_2$ needed.

(A) 22%

(B) 24%

(C) 26%

(D) 28%

(E) 31%

# CHAPTER

# *33*

# Flow Rate in Mechanical Ventilation

**EQUATION**

Minimum flow rate = $\dot{V}_E \times$ Sum of *I:E* ratio

| | | |
|---|---|---|
| Minimum flow rate | : | Minimum flow rate required to provide certain minute ventilation and *I:E* ratio, in L/min |
| $\dot{V}_E$ | : | Expired minute ventilation in L/min $(V_T \times RR)$ |
| Sum of *I:E* ratio | : | The sum of the inspiratory:expiratory *ratio* |

**EXAMPLE**

Given:    $V_T$ = 900 mL (0.9 L)

           $RR$ = 16/min

           *I:E* ratio = 1:2.5

Calculate the minimum flow rate required for the above settings.

Minimum flow rate = $\dot{V}_E \times$ Sum of *I:E* ratio

                      = $(V_T \times RR) \times$ Sum of *I:E* ratio

                      = $(0.9 \times 16) \times (1 + 2.5)$

                      = $14.4 \times 3.5$

                      = 50.4 or 50 L/min

**EXERCISE**

Given:    $V_T$ = 800 mL (0.8 L)

           $RR$ = 12/min

           *I:E* ratio = 1:3

What is the minimum flow rate needed for the above settings?

[Answer: Minimum flow rate = 38 L/min]

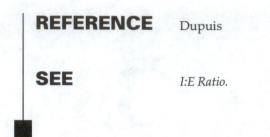

**REFERENCE**   Dupuis

**SEE**   *I:E Ratio.*

## Self-Assessment Questions

33a.   If the expired minute ventilation is 15 L/min and an *I:E* ratio of 1:2.5 is desired, what should be the *minimum* flow rate required for the above settings?

(A) 45 L/min

(B) 47 L/min

(C) 49 L/min

(D) 51 L/min

(E) 53 L/min

33b.   Given: $V_T$ = 750 mL (0.75 L), *RR* = 20/min, *I:E* ratio = 1:2.2. What should be the *minimum* flow rate required for the above settings?

(A) 40 L/min

(B) 43 L/min

(C) 48 L/min

(D) 51 L/min

(E) 53 L/min

33c.   Given: $V_T$ = 900 mL (0.9 L), *RR* = 12/min, *I:E* ratio = 1:3. What should be the *minimum* flow rate needed for these settings?

(A) 36 L/min

(B) 40 L/min

(C) 43 L/min

(D) 48 L/min

(E) 55 L/min

# *34*

# Forced Vital Capacity Tracing (FEV$_t$ and FEV$_{t\%}$)

## *NOTES*

The method to find other FEV$_t$ and FEV$_{t\%}$ measurements is the same as shown in Examples 1 and 2. For accurate results, it is extremely important to plot the points carefully and draw straight lines with a ruler.

The FEV$_{0.5}$ and FEV$_{1.0}$ (as well as FEF$_{200-1200}$) are used to assess the flow rates and disorders relating to the large airways. In patients with large airway obstruction, these values are decreased. However, poor patient effort may also lead to lower than normal results. The FEV$_{t\%}$ values are also reduced in patients with obstructive disorders.

In patients with restrictive lung disorders, essentially all FEV$_t$ measurements are decreased. However, the FEV$_{t\%}$ may be normal or increased because of the concurrent decrease in FVC. For example, when FEV$_{1.0}$ and FVC are both decreased, the FEV$_{1.0\%}$ (FEV$_{1.0}$/FVC) may show little or no change.

## EQUATION

FEV$_t$  :  Forced Expiratory Volume (timed), in liters (t is commonly expressed in 0.5, 1, 2, or 3 sec)

FEV$_{t\%}$ :  Forced Expiratory Volume (timed)/Forced Vital Capacity (FVC), in %

## NORMAL VALUES

**FEV$_t$**

FEV$_{0.5}$  =  3.1 L

FEV$_1$ =  4.2 L

FEV$_2$ =  4.6 L

FEV$_3$ =  4.8 L

The FEV$_t$ normal values are based on a 70", 20-year-old male. Since the normal predicted values are based on a person's gender, age, height, weight, smoking history, and ethnic origin, an appropriate normal table should be used to match a person's physical attributes.

**FEV$_{t\%}$**

FEV$_{0.5\%}$ =  50% to 60%

FEV$_{1\%}$    =  75% to 85%

FEV$_{2\%}$    =  94%

FEV$_{3\%}$    =  97%

FEV$_{t\%}$ expresses a person's FEV$_t$ relative to his FVC. The FEV$_{t\%}$ normal values may be accepted for all subjects regardless of gender, age, height, and other physical attributes. For clinical evaluation of lung impairments, an FEV$_{1\%}$ of 65% or less is significant and diagnostic of airway obstruction.

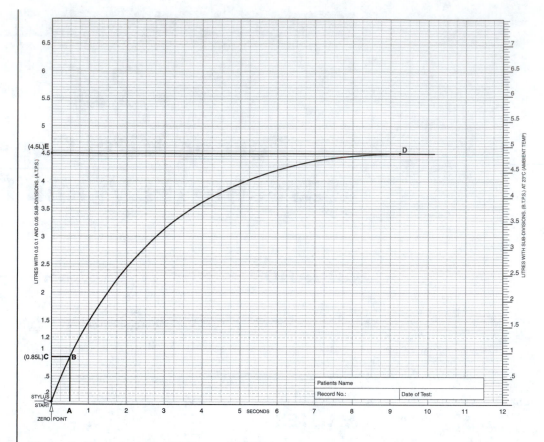

**Figure 5**  *Examples to find* FEV$_{0.5}$ *and* FEV$_{0.5\%}$.

## EXAMPLE 1

From the PFT tracing (Figure 5), find FEV$_{0.5}$.

Step 1. Along the time (x) axis, locate 0.5 sec (point A).

Step 2. From point A, draw a vertical line upward until it intersects the PFT tracing (point B).

Step 3. From point B, draw a horizontal line until it intersects the volume (y) axis (point C).

Step 4. The reading at point C (0.85 L) is the volume expired during the first 0.5 sec of the FVC maneuver.

Therefore, FEV$_{0.5}$ = 0.85 L.

## EXAMPLE 2

From the PFT tracing (Figure 5), find FEV$_{0.5\%}$. Is the result normal?

Step 1. From the PFT tracing, locate the highest point at the end of the tracing (point D).

Step 2. From point D, draw a horizontal line until it intersects the volume (y) axis (point E).

Step 3. The reading at point E (4.5 L) represents the FVC.

$$
\begin{aligned}
\text{FEV}_{0.5\%} \quad &= \quad \text{FEV}_{0.5} / \text{FVC} \\
&= \quad 0.85\,\text{L} / 4.5\,\text{L} \\
&= \quad 0.1888 \\
&= \quad 18.9\%
\end{aligned}
$$

FEV$_{0.5\%}$ of 18.9% is below normal.

**EXERCISE 1**    From the PFT tracing (Figure 6), find FEV$_1$.

[Answer: FEV$_1$ = 2.4 L] (See Figure 7)

**EXERCISE 2**    From the PFT tracing (Figure 6), find FEV$_{1\%}$. Is it normal?

[Answers: FEV$_{1\%}$ = 2.4/5.05 or 47.5%; the FEV$_{1\%}$ is lower than predicted] (See Figure 7)

**REFERENCE**    Madama

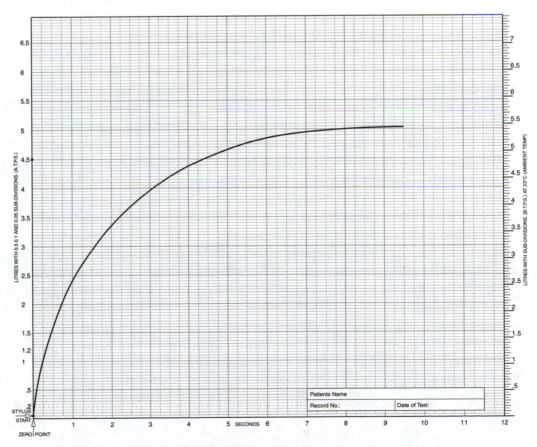

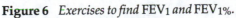

**Figure 6**  *Exercises to find* FEV$_1$ *and* FEV$_{1\%}$.

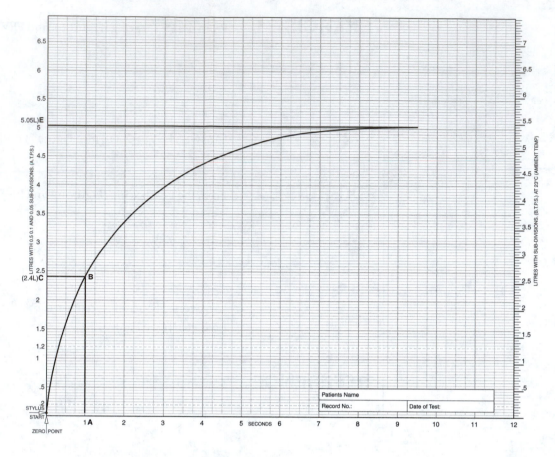

**Figure 7**   *Solutions to exercises 1 and 2 in Figure 6.*

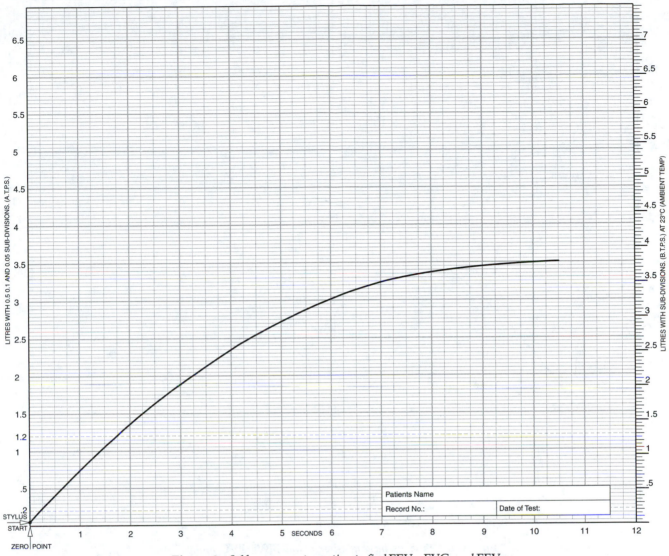

**Figure 8**  *Self-assessment question to find* FEV$_1$, FVC, *and* FEV$_{1\%}$.

## Self-Assessment Questions

34a.  From the PFT tracing (Figure 8), find FEV$_1$, FVC, and FEV$_{1\%}$. Is the FEV$_{1\%}$ normal?

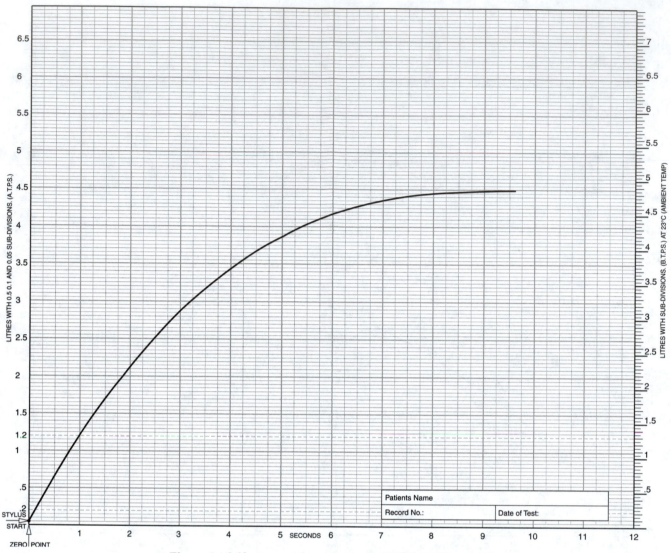

**Figure 9** *Self-assessment question to find* FEV$_2$, FVC, *and* FEV$_{2\%}$.

34b. From the PFT tracing (Figure 9), find FEV$_2$, FVC, and FEV$_{2\%}$. Is the FEV$_{2\%}$ normal?

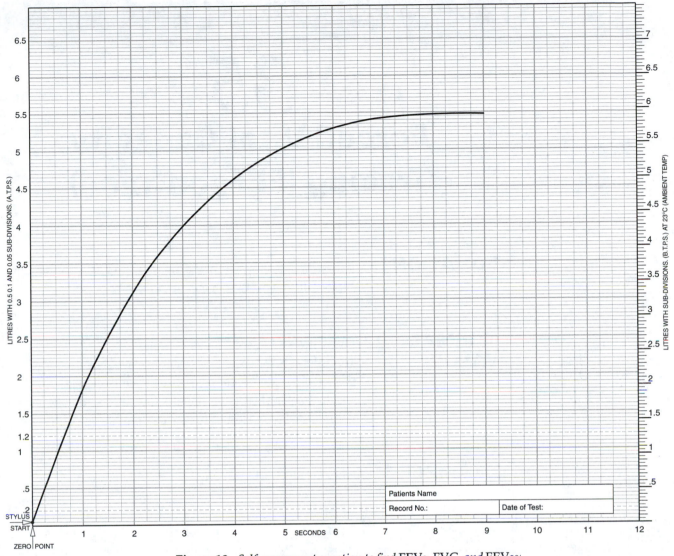

**Figure 10** *Self-assessment question to find* FEV$_3$, FVC, *and* FEV$_3$%.

34c. From the PFT tracing (Figure 10), find FEV$_3$, FVC, and FEV$_3$%. Is the FEV$_3$% normal?

# 35

# Forced Vital Capacity Tracing (FEF$_{200}$-1200)

## NOTES

The FEF$_{200-1200}$ measurement is dependent on the slope derived from the PFT tracing. A steep PFT tracing results in a higher FEF$_{200-1200}$ measurement. The method to plot the slopes from other PFT tracings is the same as shown in Example 1. For accurate results, it is extremely important to plot the points accurately and draw straight lines with a ruler.

The FEF$_{200-1200}$ (as well as FEV$_{0.5}$ and FEV$_{1.0}$) is used to assess the flow rates and disorders relating to the large airways. In patients with large airway obstruction, the FEF$_{200-1200}$ values are usually decreased. However, poor patient effort may also lead to lower than normal results.

## EQUATION

FEF$_{200-1200}$  :  Flow rate of the initial 200 to 1200 mL of volume expired during the FVC maneuver, in L/sec.

## NORMAL VALUE

FEF$_{200-1200}$ = 8.7 L/sec
This value is based on a 70", 20-year-old male. Since the normal predicted values are based on a person's gender, age, height, weight, smoking history, and ethnic origin, an appropriate normal table should be used to match a person's physical attributes.

## EXAMPLE 1

From the PFT tracing (Figure 11), find FEF$_{200-1200}$.

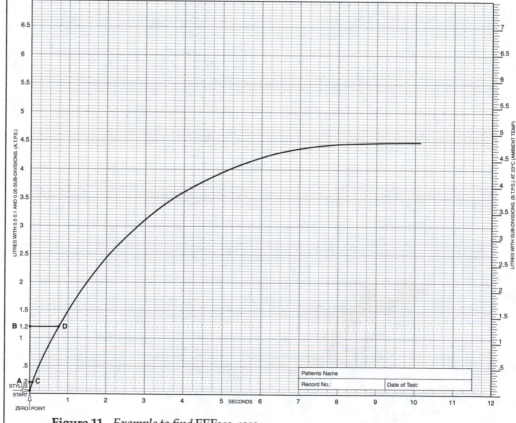

**Figure 11** *Example to find* FEF$_{200-1200}$.

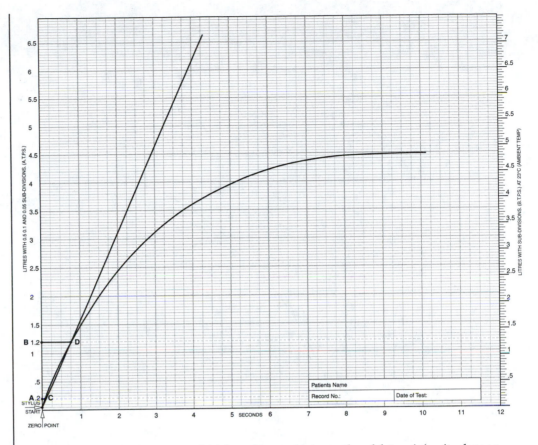

**Figure 12** *Locating the 0.2 L and 1.2 L markings on spirograph and determining its slope on graph paper.*

Figure 12    Step 1. Along the volume (y) axis, locate 0.2 L (point A) and 1.2 L (point B).

Step 2. From point A, draw a horizontal line until it intersects the PFT tracing (point C). Do the same from point B until the line intersects the PFT tracing (point D).

Step 3. Use a ruler to draw a straight line connecting points C and D. Extend this straight line to top of graph paper. This is the FEF$_{200-1200}$ SLOPE.

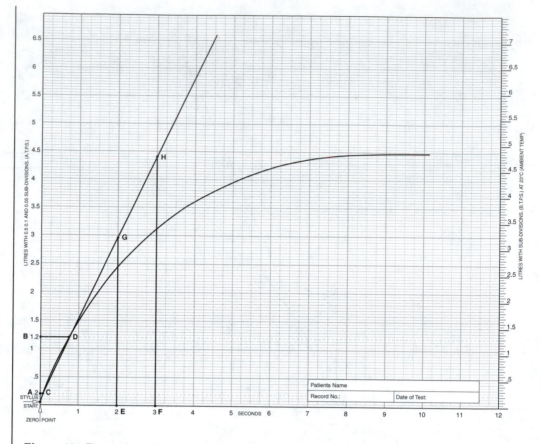

**Figure 13**   *Determining the one-second interval on graph paper (points E, F) and spirograph tracing (points G, H).*

Figure 13   Step 4.  Along the time (x) axis, select two adjacent second-lines and mark them points E and F. (In the example shown, the 2nd and 3rd second-lines are used. One may use the 3rd and 4th second-lines. The result would be identical since these two sets of adjacent lines intersect the same slope).

Step 5.  From point E, follow the second line vertically until it intersects the slope (point G). Do the same from point F until it intersects the slope (point H).

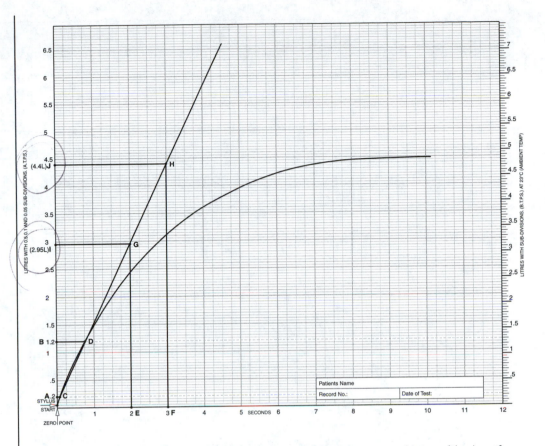

**Figure 14** *Determining the volume (L) that corresponds to the one-second interval (sec) on the slope. The unit of this reading is L/sec.*

Figure 14    Step 6. From point G, draw a horizontal line until it intersects the volume (y) axis (point I). Do the same from point H until it intersects the volume (y) axis (point J).

Step 7. The difference between the volume readings taken at points I and J represents the flow rate of the initial 200 to 1200 mL of volume expired during the FVC maneuver.

$$\text{FEF}_{200\text{-}1200} = (4.4\,\text{L} - 2.95\,\text{L})/\text{sec}$$
$$= 1.45\,\text{L}/\text{sec}$$

## EXERCISE

From the PFT tracing (Figure 15), find $\text{FEF}_{200\text{-}1200}$.

[Answer: $\text{FEF}_{200\text{-}1200} = (6.9\,\text{L} - 3.5\,\text{L})/\text{sec}$ or $3.4\,\text{L}/\text{sec}$] (See Figure 16)

## REFERENCE

Madama

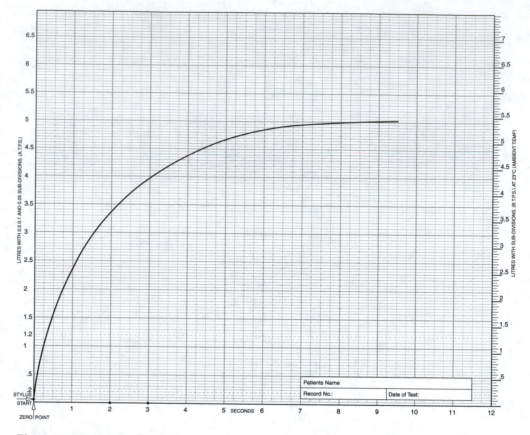

**Figure 15** *Exercise to find* FEF$_{200-1200}$.

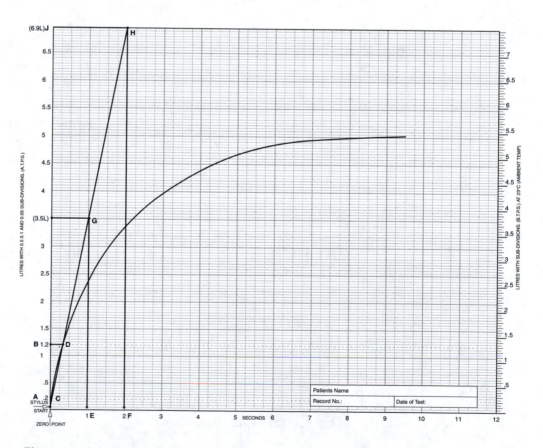

**Figure 16** *Solution to exercise in Figure 15.*

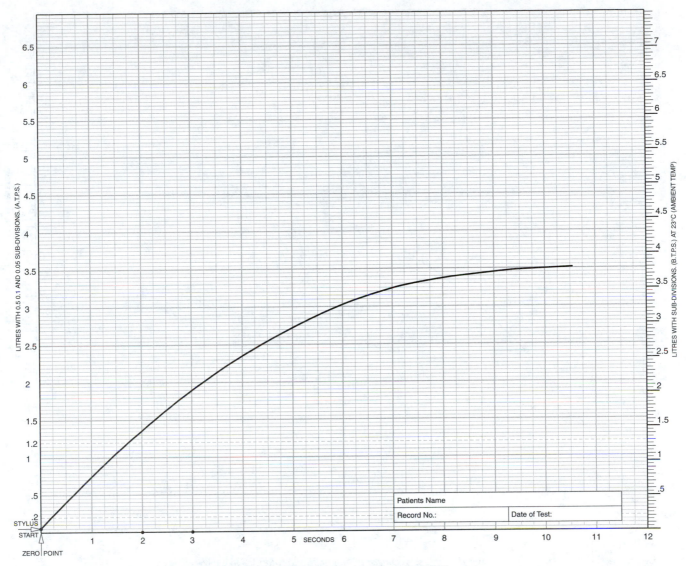

**Figure 17**   *Self-assessment question 35a to find* FEF$_{200-1200}$.

## Self-Assessment Questions

35a.   From the PFT tracing (Figure 17), find FEF$_{200-1200}$.

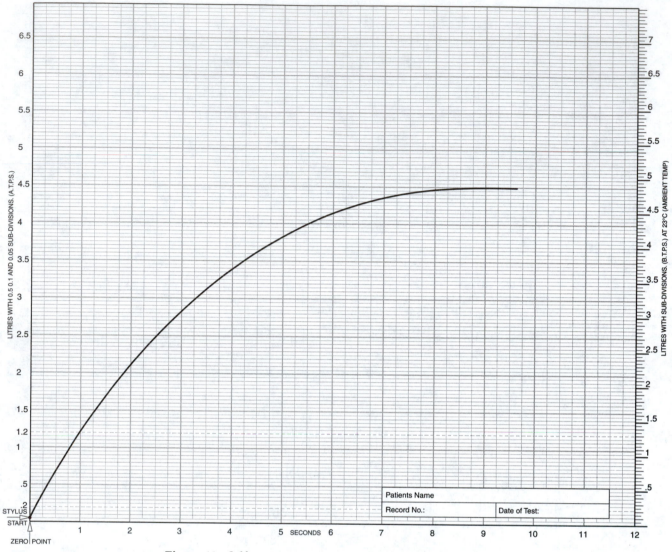

**Figure 18** *Self-assessment question 35b to find* FEF$_{200-1200}$.

35b.  From the PFT tracing (Figure 18), find FEF$_{200-1200}$.

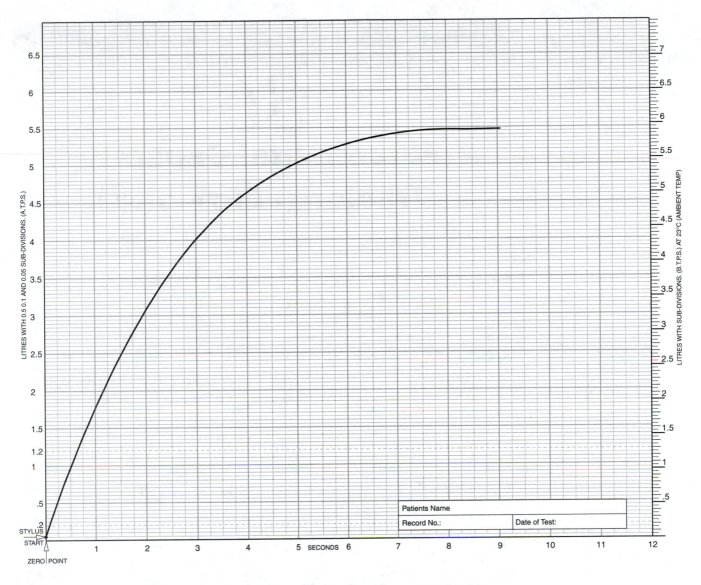

*Figure 19   Self-assessment question 35c to find* FEF$_{200-1200}$.

35c.   From the PFT tracing (Figure 19), find FEF$_{200-1200}$.

# CHAPTER

# *36*
# Forced Vital Capacity Tracing (FEF25-75%)

## *NOTES*

The method to plot the FEF25-75% slopes from other PFT tracings is the same as shown in Example 1. For accurate results, it is extremely important to locate and plot the points carefully and draw straight lines using a ruler.

The FEF25-75% (as well as FEV2) is used to assess the flow rates and disorders relating to the smaller bronchi and larger bronchioles. In patients with early airway obstruction, the FEF25-75% values are usually decreased. Patient effort has minimal effect on the FEF25-75% measurements.

## EQUATION

FEF25-75% :   Flow rate of the middle 50% of the volume expired during the FVC maneuver, in L/sec.

## NORMAL VALUES

FEF25-75% = 5.2 L/sec

This value is based on a 70", 20-year-old male. Since the normal predicted values are based on a person's gender, age, height, weight, smoking history, and ethnic origin, an appropriate normal table should be used to match a person's physical attributes.

## EXAMPLE 1

From the PFT tracing (Figure 20), find FEF25-75%.

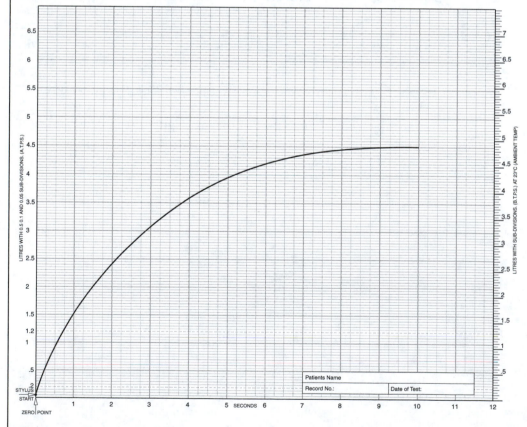

**Figure 20**   *Example to find* FEF25–75%.

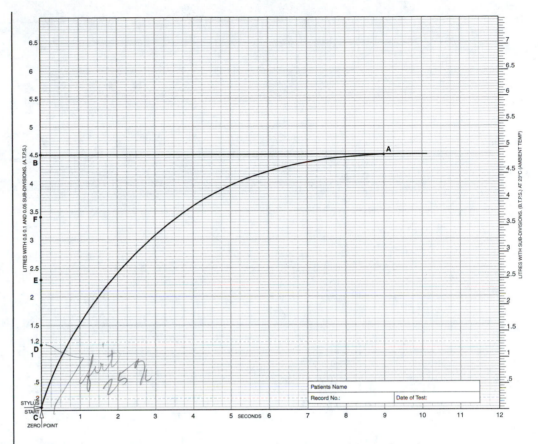

**Figure 21**  *Determining the FVC and the four 25% segments of the FVC tracing.*

Figure 21   Step 1. From the PFT tracing, locate the highest point at the end of the tracing (point A).

Step 2. From point A, draw a horizontal line until it intersects the volume (y) axis (point B).

Step 3. The difference between point B and the starting point C (4.5 L) represents the FVC.

Step 4. Divide the 4.5 L by 4 to obtain four equal segments. Plot the points D, E, F on the volume (y) axis to divide segment BC into 4 equal segments.

The volume between points C and D represents the first 25% of the volume expired during the FVC maneuver. The volume between points D and F represents the middle 50% of the expired volume. The volume between points B and F represents the last 25% of the expired volume.

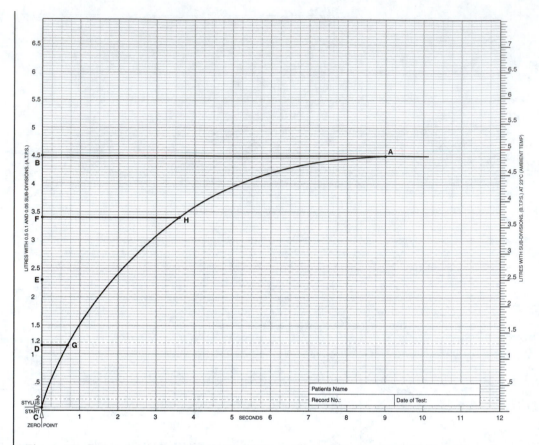

**Figure 22** *Determining the middle 50% of FVC on the graph paper (points D, F) and the spirograph (points G, H).*

Figure 22   Step 5. From point D, draw a horizontal line until it intersects the PFT tracing (point G). Do the same from point F until the line intersects the PFT tracing (point H).

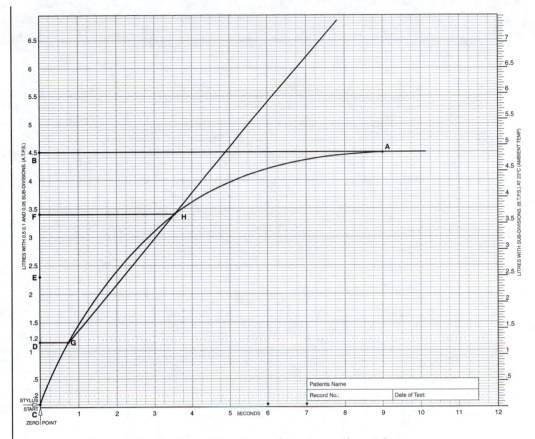

**Figure 23**   *Determining the slope of the spirograph tracing on the graph paper.*

Figure 23   Step 6. Use a ruler to draw a straight line joining points G and H. Extend this straight line to top of graph paper. This is the SLOPE for this FEF$_{25-75\%}$ determination.

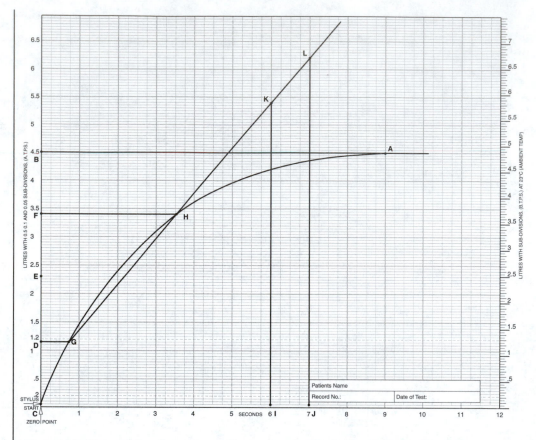

**Figure 24** *Determining the one-second interval on the graph paper (points I, J) and the spiro-graph tracing (points K, L).*

Figure 24   Step 7.  Along the time (x) axis, select two adjacent second-lines and mark them points I and J. (In the example shown, the 6th and 7th second-lines are used. One may wish to use two other adjacent second-lines as long as the resulting drawings do not overlap or become too close to other existing lines. The result would be identical since any two adjacent lines intersect the same slope.)

Step 8.  From point I, follow the second line vertically until it intersects the slope (point K). Do the same from point J until it intersects the slope (point L).

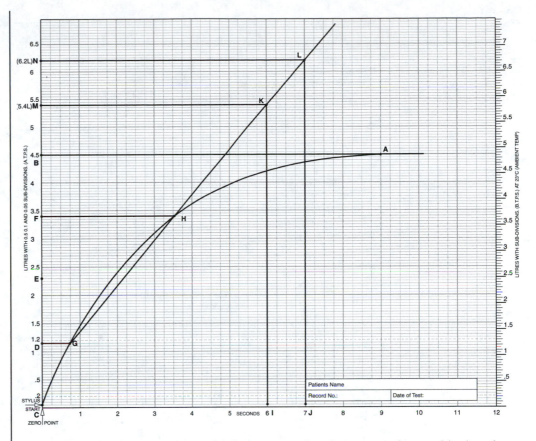

**Figure 25**   *Determining the volume (L) that corresponds to the one-second interval (sec) on the slope. The unit of this reading is L/sec.*

Figure 25   Step 9. From point K, draw a horizontal line until it intersects the volume (y) axis (point M). Do the same from point L until it intersects the volume (y) axis (point N).

Step 10.   The difference between the volume readings taken at points N and M represents the flow rate of the middle 50% of volume expired during the FVC maneuver.

$$\text{FEF}_{25\text{-}75\%} = (6.2 \text{ L} - 5.4 \text{ L})/\text{sec}$$
$$= 0.8 \text{ L}/\text{sec}$$

## EXERCISE

From the PFT tracing (Figure 26), find $\text{FEF}_{25\text{-}75\%}$.

[Answer: $\text{FEF}_{25\text{-}75\%} = (6.3 \text{ L} - 5.25 \text{ L})/\text{sec}$ or 1.05 L/sec] (See Figure 27)

## REFERENCE

Madama

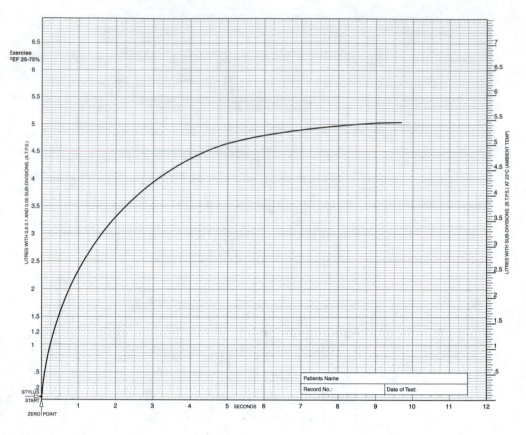

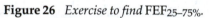

**Figure 26** *Exercise to find* FEF25–75%.

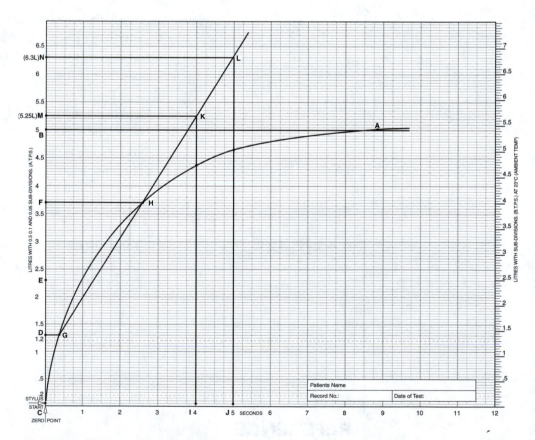

**Figure 27** *Solutions to exercise in Figure 26.*

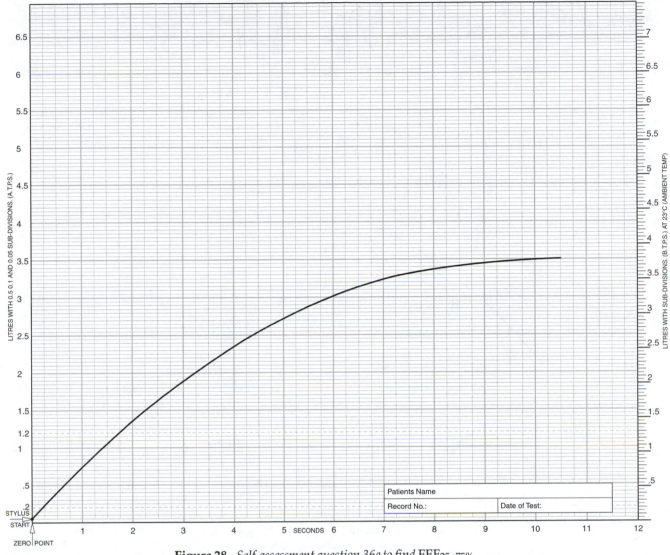

**Figure 28** *Self-assessment question 36a to find* FEF25–75%.

# Self-Assessment Questions

36a. From the PFT tracing (Figure 28), find FEF25-75%.

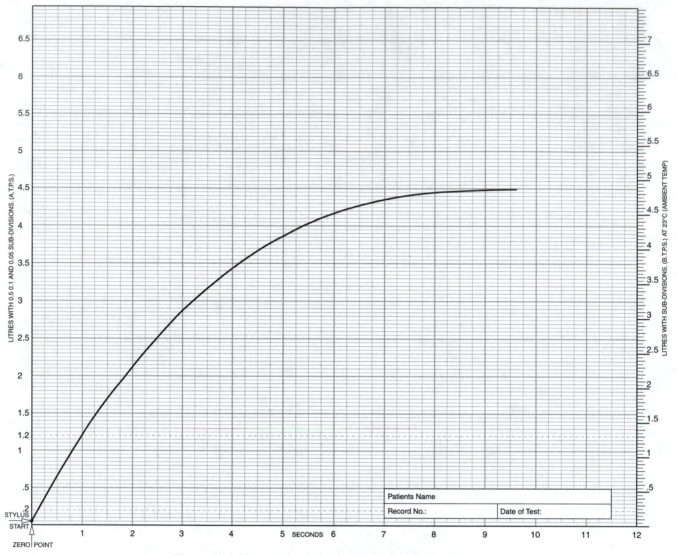

**Figure 29** *Self-assessment question 36b to find* FEF$_{25-75\%}$.

36b. From the PFT tracing (Figure 29), find FEF$_{25-75\%}$.

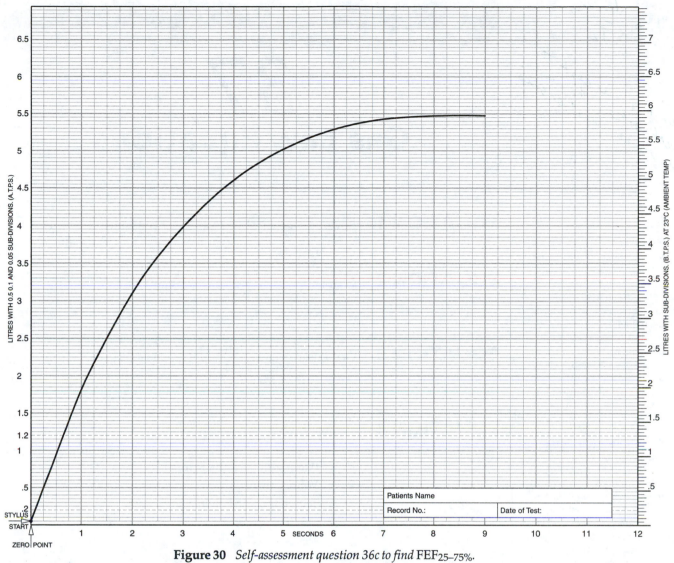

**Figure 30**  *Self-assessment question 36c to find* FEF25–75%.

36c.   From the PFT tracing (Figure 30), find FEF25-75%.

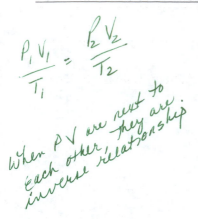

$$\frac{P_1 V_1}{T_1} = \frac{P_2 V_2}{T_2}$$

*When P V are next to each other, they are inverse relationship*

# 37
# Gas Law Equations

## NOTES

**Boyle's law (Robert Boyle)**
The pressure and volume are inversely related. For example, a diver upon ascending to the surface (decreasing barometric pressure) must exhale more than he inhales to rid of the increasing lung volume. In respiratory care, this relationship between pressure and volume can be used to measure indirectly the functional residual capacity or the residual volume.

**Charles' law (Jacques Charles)**
The volume and absolute temperature (in kelvins) are directly related. Charles' law is most commonly used in respiratory care to correct lung volumes and flow rates measured at room temperature, to that measured at body temperature.**

**Gay-Lussac's law (Joseph Gay-Lussac)**
The pressure and temperature are directly related. For example, the air pressure in a car tire increases as the surrounding temperature increases, and vice versa.

**Combined Gas Law**
This is also called the modified Ideal Gas Law. The Combined Gas Law accounts for all three factors (*P, V, T*) affecting gas behaviors. This equation is especially useful when precise measurements are required.

**EQUATION 1** Boyle's law: $P_1 \times V_1 = P_2 \times V_2$ ($T$ constant)

**EQUATION 2** Charles' law: $\frac{V_1}{T_1} = \frac{V_2}{T_2}$ (P constant)

**EQUATION 3** Gay-Lussac's Law: $\frac{P_1}{T_1} = \frac{P_2}{T_2}$ (V constant)

**EQUATION 4** Combined Gas Law: $\frac{P_1 \times V_1}{T_1} = \frac{P_2 \times V_2}{T_2}$

$P$ : Barometric pressure in mm Hg
$V$ : Volume in mL
$T$ : Temperature in kelvins*
1 : Original values
2 : New values

**EXAMPLE** SEE: Gas Volume Corrections.

**EXERCISE** $P_1 \times V_1 = P_2 \times V_2$ is the _____ law.

$\frac{P_1}{T_1} = \frac{P_2}{T_2}$ is the _____ law.

$\frac{V_1}{T_1} = \frac{V_2}{T_2}$ is the _____ law.

Write the Combined Gas Law equation _____

**REFERENCE** Scanlan

**SEE** *Gas Volume Corrections.*

*See: Temperature Conversion (˚C to K).
**ATPS to BTPS.

## Self-Assessment Questions

*MATCHING:* Match the gas laws with their appropriate equations. Use only *three* of the answers in Column II.

| Column I | Column II |
|---|---|
| 37a. Gay-Lussac's law | (A) $P_1V_1 = P_2V_2$ |
| 37b. Charles' law | (B) $\dfrac{P_1}{V_1} = \dfrac{P_2}{V_2}$ |
| 37c. Boyle's law | (C) $\dfrac{V_1}{T_1} = \dfrac{V_2}{T_2}$ |
| | (D) $\dfrac{P_1}{T_1} = \dfrac{P_2}{T_2}$ |
| | (E) $\dfrac{T_1}{V_1} = \dfrac{T_2}{V_2}$ |

37d. $P_1 \times V_1 = P_2 \times V_2$ is which of the following gas laws?

(A) Gay-Lussac's

(B) Charles'

(C) Boyle's

(D) Combined

(E) Henry's

37e. Charles' law is represented by the equation

(A) $P_1 \times V_1 = P_2 \times V_2$

(B) $\dfrac{P_1}{T_1} = \dfrac{P_2}{T_2}$

(C) $\dfrac{V_1}{T_1} = \dfrac{V_2}{T_2}$

(D) $\dfrac{P_1}{V_1} = \dfrac{P_2}{V_2}$

(E) $P_1 \times T_1 = P_2 \times T_2$

37f. Gay-Lussac's law is represented by the equation

(A) $P_1 \times V_1 = P_2 \times V_2$

(B) $\dfrac{P_1}{T_1} = \dfrac{P_2}{T_2}$

(C) $\dfrac{V_1}{T_1} = \dfrac{V_2}{T_2}$

(D) $\dfrac{P_1}{V_1} = \dfrac{P_2}{V_2}$

(E) $P_1 \times T_1 = P_2 \times T_2$

37g. According to Charles' law, at constant _____ , the gas volume varies directly with the _____ .

(A) pressure; diffusion rate

(B) temperature; pressure

(C) pressure; temperature

(D) temperature; solubility

(E) pressure; content

37h. Correction of lung volumes and flow rates from ATPS to BTPS is based on

(A) Gay-Lussac's law

(B) Charles; law

(C) Boyle's law

(D) the Bohr effect

(E) the Haldane effect

37i. In using the gas law equations, the temperature must first be converted to

(A) degrees Celsius

(B) degrees Fahrenheit

(C) kelvins

(D) degrees Centigrade

(E) absolute zero

37j. Which gas law states that at a constant temperature the gas volume varies inversely with the pressure?

(A) Charles' law

(B) Dalton's law

(C) Boyle's law

(D) Ideal Gas Law

(E) Gay-Lussac's law

# CHAPTER

# *38*

# Gas Volume Corrections

## EQUATION

Since $\dfrac{P_1 \times V_1}{T_1} = \dfrac{P_2 \times V_2}{T_2}$ (Combined Gas Law),

$$V_2 = \dfrac{P_1 \times V_1 \times T_2}{T_1 \times P_2}$$

$V_2$ : New gas volume in mL
$P_1$ : Original pressure $(P_B - PH_2O)$
$V_1$ : Original gas volume in mL
$T_2$ : New temperature in kelvins (K)
$T_1$ : Original temperature in kelvins (K)
$P_2$ : New pressure $(P_B - PH_2O)$

### NOTES

Before using these equations for gas volume corrections, the temperature must be converted to the Kelvin (K) temperature scale.

For gas volume correction problems involving *dry* gas, delete $PH_2O$ and use only $P_B$.

For gas correction problems involving the same pressure, delete $P_1$ and $P_2$ from the Combined Gas Law equation and it becomes:

> Charles' law: $\dfrac{V_1}{T_1} = \dfrac{V_2}{T_2}$

To find new volume ($V_2$) or new temperature ($T_2$):

> $V_2 = \dfrac{V_1 \times T_2}{T_1}$ or $T_2 = \dfrac{V_2 \times T_1}{V_1}$

For gas correction problems involving the same temperature, delete $T_1$ and $T_2$ from the Combined Gas Law equation and it becomes:

> Boyle's law: $P_1 \times V_1 = P_2 \times V_2$

To find new volume ($V_2$) or new pressure ($P_2$):

> $V_2 = \dfrac{P_1 \times V_1}{P_2}$ or $P_2 = \dfrac{P_1 \times V_1}{V_2}$

## EXAMPLE 1

Given: 100 mL of saturated gas volume measured at 25 °C and 750 mm Hg.

Find the new saturated gas volume measured at 37 °C and 760 mm Hg.

At 25 °C, $PH_2O = 23.8$ mm Hg (Appendix I).

$P_1 = P_B1 - PH_2O = (750 - 23.8)$ mm Hg $= 726.2$ mm Hg

At 37 °C, $PH_2O = 47$ mm Hg (Appendix I).

$P_2 = P_B2 - PH_2O = (760 - 47)$ mm Hg $= 713$ mm Hg

$V_1 = 100$ mL

$T_1 = 25\,°C = (25 + 273)K = 298\ K$

$T_2 = 37\,°C = (37 + 273)K = 310\ K$

$V_2 = \dfrac{P_1 \times V_1 \times T_2}{T_1 \times P_2}$

$= \dfrac{726.2 \times 100 \times 310}{298 \times 713}$

$= \dfrac{22,512,200}{212,474}$

$= 105.95$ or 106 mL

## EXAMPLE 2

A saturated tidal volume of 500 mL was measured at 24 °C and 750 mm Hg. Find the new saturated gas volume corrected to 37 °C and 760 mm Hg.

Given: At 24 °C, $PH_2O$ = 22.4 mm Hg (Appendix I)

At 37 °C, $PH_2O$ = 47 mm Hg (Appendix I)

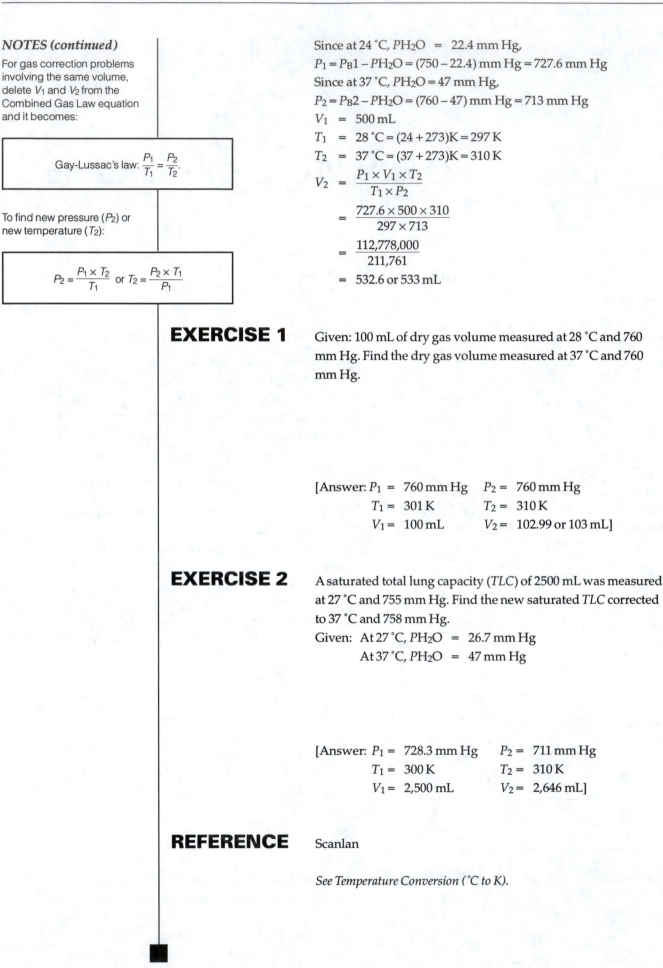

*NOTES (continued)*

For gas correction problems involving the same volume, delete $V_1$ and $V_2$ from the Combined Gas Law equation and it becomes:

Gay-Lussac's law: $\dfrac{P_1}{T_1} = \dfrac{P_2}{T_2}$.

To find new pressure ($P_2$) or new temperature ($T_2$):

$$P_2 = \frac{P_1 \times T_2}{T_1} \quad \text{or} \quad T_2 = \frac{P_2 \times T_1}{P_1}$$

Since at 24 °C, $PH_2O$ = 22.4 mm Hg,

$P_1 = P_B1 - PH_2O = (750 - 22.4)$ mm Hg = 727.6 mm Hg

Since at 37 °C, $PH_2O$ = 47 mm Hg,

$P_2 = P_B2 - PH_2O = (760 - 47)$ mm Hg = 713 mm Hg

$V_1$ = 500 mL

$T_1$ = 28 °C = (24 + 273)K = 297 K

$T_2$ = 37 °C = (37 + 273)K = 310 K

$$V_2 = \frac{P_1 \times V_1 \times T_2}{T_1 \times P_2}$$

$$= \frac{727.6 \times 500 \times 310}{297 \times 713}$$

$$= \frac{112{,}778{,}000}{211{,}761}$$

= 532.6 or 533 mL

## EXERCISE 1

Given: 100 mL of dry gas volume measured at 28 °C and 760 mm Hg. Find the dry gas volume measured at 37 °C and 760 mm Hg.

[Answer: $P_1$ = 760 mm Hg    $P_2$ = 760 mm Hg

        $T_1$ = 301 K       $T_2$ = 310 K

        $V_1$ = 100 mL     $V_2$ = 102.99 or 103 mL]

## EXERCISE 2

A saturated total lung capacity (*TLC*) of 2500 mL was measured at 27 °C and 755 mm Hg. Find the new saturated *TLC* corrected to 37 °C and 758 mm Hg.

Given:   At 27 °C, $PH_2O$ = 26.7 mm Hg

        At 37 °C, $PH_2O$ = 47 mm Hg

[Answer: $P_1$ = 728.3 mm Hg    $P_2$ = 711 mm Hg

        $T_1$ = 300 K       $T_2$ = 310 K

        $V_1$ = 2,500 mL    $V_2$ = 2,646 mL]

## REFERENCE

Scanlan

*See Temperature Conversion (°C to K).*

## Self-Assessment Questions

38a. Given:

$P_1 = 760$ mm Hg    $P_2 = 755$ mm Hg
$T_1 = 300$ K    $T_2 = 310$ K
$V_1 = 800$ mL

Find $V_2$ using the Combined Gas Law.

(A) 809 mL

(B) 814 mL

(C) 825 mL

(D) 832 mL

(E) 840 mL

38b. A saturated gas sample of 1000 mL was measured at 28 °C and 750 mm Hg. Find the new saturated gas volume corrected to 37 °C and 760 mm Hg. (At 28 °C, $PH_2O$ = 28.3 mm Hg; at 37 °C, $PH_2O$ = 47 mm Hg.)

(A) 1042 mL

(B) 1016 mL

(C) 995 mL

(D) 987 mL

(E) 980 mL

38c. The forced vital capacity (*FVC*) of a patient measured at 26 °C and 760 mm Hg is 3000 mL. Find the new *FVC* corrected to 37 °C and 758 mm Hg. (At 26 °C, $PH_2O$ = 25.2 mm Hg; at 37 °C, $PH_2O$ = 47 mm Hg.)

(A) 3119 mL

(B) 3161 mL

(C) 3203 mL

(D) 3215 mL

(E) 3258 mL

38d. Given the following information: measured tidal volume ($V_T$) = 670 mL; temperature and pressure under which $V_T$ was obtained = 27 °C and 758 mm Hg. Calculated the corrected $V_T$ at 37 °C and 760 mm Hg. (At 27 °C, $PH_2O$ = 26.7 mm Hg; at 37 °C, $PH_2O$ = 47 mm Hg.)

(A) 649 mL

(B) 665 mL

(C) 680 mL

(D) 691 mL

(E) 710 mL

# CHAPTER

# 39

# Graham's Law of Diffusion Coefficient

## EQUATION

$$D = \frac{\text{Sol. Coeff.}}{\sqrt{gmw}}$$

| | | |
|---|---|---|
| $D$ | : | Diffusion coefficient |
| Sol. Coeff. | : | Solubility coefficient of gas |
| $\sqrt{gmw}$ | : | Square root of gram molecular weight of gas |

## EXAMPLE

The diffusion coefficient of carbon dioxide is 19 times $\left(\dfrac{0.077}{0.004}\right)$ greater than that of oxygen. This is shown below by computing the diffusion coefficient of each gas.

$$D_{\text{carbon dioxide}} = \frac{0.510}{\sqrt{44}} \qquad D_{\text{oxygen}} = \frac{0.023}{\sqrt{32}}$$

$$= \frac{0.510}{6.633} \qquad\qquad = \frac{0.023}{5.657}$$

$$= 0.077 \qquad\qquad\quad = 0.004$$

The difference in diffusion coefficient between carbon dioxide and oxygen explains why a small carbon dioxide pressure gradient of 6 mm Hg ($P_{\bar{v}}CO_2$ 46 mm Hg – $P_ACO_2$ 40 mm Hg) across the alveolar-capillary membrane is sufficient for carbon dioxide elimination. On the other hand, a much larger pressure gradient of 60 mm Hg ($P_AO_2$ 100 mm Hg – $P_{\bar{v}}O_2$ 40 mm Hg) is needed for oxygen uptake by the pulmonary capillaries.

## REFERENCE

Scanlan

## SEE

*Fick's Law of Diffusion.*

### NOTES

In 1833, the Scottish inorganic and physical chemist Thomas Graham proposed Graham's law, which states that the rate of gas diffusion is inversely proportional to the square root of its gram molecular weight. The solubility coefficient in the equation is added for calculation of the diffusion coefficient.

In pulmonary disorders that impair the lung's diffusion rate, hypoxia is usually a more difficult situation to correct than is hypercapnia. This is due to the low diffusion coefficient of oxygen.

## Self-Assessment Questions

39a.  The diffusion coefficient of a gas is described by

(A) Charles' law

(B) Gay-Lussac's law

(C) Graham's law

(D) Henry's law

(E) Dalton's law

39b.  The diffusion coefficient of a gas is _____ related to its solubility coefficient and _____ related to the square root of its gram molecular weight.

(A) directly; inversely

(B) directly; directly

(C) inversely; inversely

(D) inversely; directly

(E) not; inversely

39c.  The diffusion coefficient of carbon dioxide is about _____ times higher than that of oxygen. For this reason, hypoxia is _____ to treat than hypercapnia in the absence of airway obstruction.

(A) 210; more difficult

(B) 30; more difficult

(C) 30; easier

(D) 19; easier

(E) 19; more difficult

CHAPTER

# *40*
# Helium/Oxygen (He/O₂) Flow Rate Conversion

*NOTES*

A conversion factor (e.g., 1.8 or 1.6) must be used if an oxygen flowmeter is used to regulate a helium/oxygen gas mixture. This factor provides a more accurate flow rate because of the lower density of a helium/oxygen mixture.

The conversion factors are 1.8 for an 80%He/20%O₂ mixture and 1.6 for a 70%He/30%O₂ mixture.

Helium/oxygen mixture is sometimes used in patients with diffuse airway obstruction or obstruction caused by excessive secretions. It provides relief from hypoxia because a helium/oxygen mixture has a higher diffusion rate than oxygen or air alone.

Because of the high diffusion rate of a helium/oxygen mixture, a closely fitted oxygen delivering device such as a nonrebreathing mask should be used.

## EQUATION 1

Actual flow rate of 80%He / 20%O₂ = Flow rate × 1.8

## Equation 2

Actual flow rate of 70%He / 30%O₂ = Flow rate × 1.6

## EXAMPLE

Given: A gas mixture of 70%He / 30%O₂ is running at a flow rate of 10 L / min with an oxygen flowmeter. What is the actual flow rate of this He / O₂ gas mixture?

$$
\begin{aligned}
\text{Actual flow rate of 70\%He / 30\%O}_2 \ &= \ \text{Flow rate} \times 1.6 \\
&= \ 10 \text{ L / min} \times 1.6 \\
&= \ 16 \text{ L / min}
\end{aligned}
$$

## EXERCISE

Given: An oxygen flowmeter is being used to administer 8 L / min of an 80%He / 20%O₂ gas mixture.
What is the actual flow rate of this gas mixture?

[Answer: Flow rate = 14.4 L / min]

## REFERENCE

Scanlan

# Self-Assessment Questions

40a. Given: a gas mixture of 70%He/30%O₂ is running at a flow rate of 5 L/min on an oxygen flowmeter. What is the actual flow rate of this gas mixture?

(A) 4 L/min

(B) 6 L/min

(C) 7 L/min

(D) 8 L/min

(E) 11 L/min

40b. An oxygen flowmeter is being used to regulate a gas mixture of 70%He/30%O₂. If the flow rate is set at 6 L/min, what is the actual flow rate of this He/O₂ gas mixture?

(A) 12 L/min

(B) 10.8 L/min

(C) 9.6 L/min

(D) 8.3 L/min

(E) 6 L/min

40c. Calculate the actual flow rate if an 80%He/20%O₂ gas mixture is running at 5 L/min on an oxygen flow meter.

(A) 5 L/min

(B) 6 L/min

(C) 7 L/min

(D) 8 L/min

(E) 9 L/min

40d. If an oxygen flowmeter is used to regulate an 80%He/20%O₂ gas mixture and a flow rate of 10 L/min is desired, what should be the flow rate set on the oxygen flow meter?

(A) 4.5 L/min

(B) 5.6 L/min

(C) 6.3 L/min

(D) 7.7 L/min

(E) 10 L/min

# CHAPTER

# *41*
# Humidity Deficit

*NOTES*

In the humidity deficit equation, 43.9 mg/L represents the maximum humidity capacity at body temperature. Humidity deficit is dependent on the humidity content of the inspired air. A higher humidity content in the inspired air gives a lower humidity deficit. On the other hand, a lower humidity content means a higher humidity deficit.

Humidifiers and aerosol nebulizers are used to increase the humidity content of the inspired air, and thus a lower humidity deficit.

## EQUATION

HD = Capacity – Content

HD             :    Humidity deficit in mg/L
Capacity   :    Maximum amount of water the alveolar air can
                      hold at body temperature (43.9 mg/L at 37 °C).
                      Also known as maximum absolute humidity
Content     :    Humidity content of inspired air; actual humidity
                      or absolute humidity

## EXAMPLE

Calculate the humidity deficit at body temperature if the inspired air has a humidity content of 26 mg/L.
Since the humidity capacity at body temperature is 43.9 mg/L (Appendix I),

HD =   Capacity – Content
    =   43.9 – 26
    =   17.9 or 18 mg/L

## EXERCISE 1

Calculate the humidity deficit if the humidity content is 34 mg/L and capacity is 43.9 mg/L.

[Answer: HD = 9.9 or 10 mg/L]

## EXERCISE 2

Use Appendix I to find the humidity capacity at normal body temperature (37 °C) and calculate the humidity deficit when the inspired air has a humidity content of 32 mg/L.

[Answer: HD = 11.9 or 12 mg/L]

**REFERENCE**    Scanlan

**SEE**    *Appendix I: Humidity Capacity of Saturated Gas at Selected Temperatures.*

## Self-Assessment Questions

41a. What is the humidity deficit at body temperature if the humidity content of inspired air is 22 mg/L? (Humidity capacity at 37 °C = 43.9 mg/L.)

(A) 11 mg/L

(B) 22 mg/L

(C) 30 mg/L

(D) 37 mg/L

(E) 44 mg/L

41b. Calculate the humidity deficit at body temperature if the inspired air has a humidity content of 27 mg/L and the humidity capacity at 37 °C is 43.9 mg/L.

(A) 17 mg/L

(B) 27 mg/L

(C) 32 mg/L

(D) 37 mg/L

(E) 44 mg/L

# CHAPTER

# *42*

# *I:E* Ratio

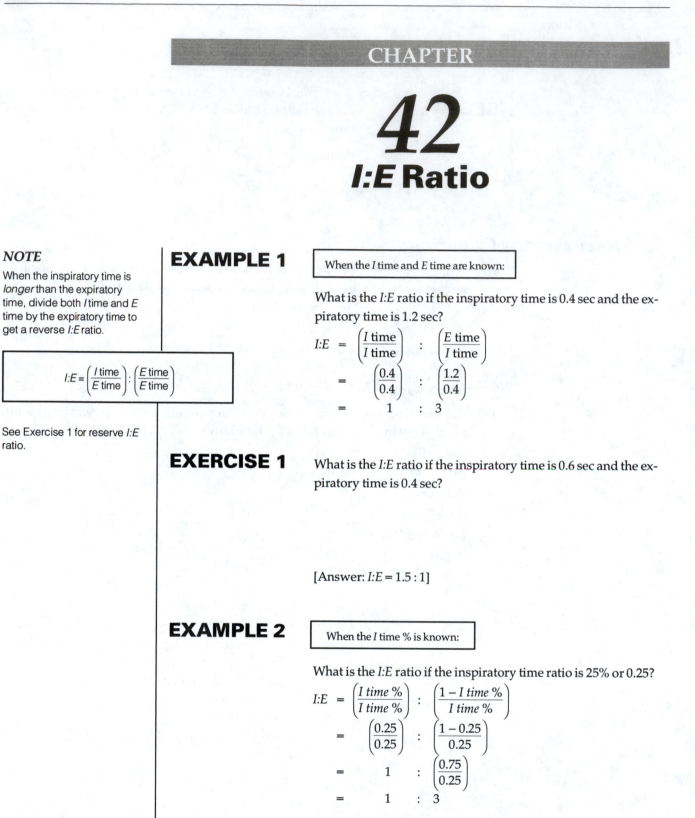

**NOTE**

When the inspiratory time is *longer* than the expiratory time, divide both *I* time and *E* time by the expiratory time to get a reverse *I:E* ratio.

$$I:E = \left( \frac{I \text{ time}}{E \text{ time}} \right) : \left( \frac{E \text{ time}}{E \text{ time}} \right)$$

See Exercise 1 for reserve *I:E* ratio.

## EXAMPLE 1

When the *I* time and *E* time are known:

What is the *I:E* ratio if the inspiratory time is 0.4 sec and the expiratory time is 1.2 sec?

$$
\begin{aligned}
I:E \ &= \ \left( \frac{I \text{ time}}{I \text{ time}} \right) \ : \ \left( \frac{E \text{ time}}{I \text{ time}} \right) \\
&= \ \left( \frac{0.4}{0.4} \right) \ : \ \left( \frac{1.2}{0.4} \right) \\
&= \ \ \ 1 \ \ \ : \ \ 3
\end{aligned}
$$

## EXERCISE 1

What is the *I:E* ratio if the inspiratory time is 0.6 sec and the expiratory time is 0.4 sec?

[Answer: *I:E* = 1.5 : 1]

## EXAMPLE 2

When the *I* time % is known:

What is the *I:E* ratio if the inspiratory time ratio is 25% or 0.25?

$$
\begin{aligned}
I:E \ &= \ \left( \frac{I \text{ time \%}}{I \text{ time \%}} \right) \ : \ \left( \frac{1 - I \text{ time \%}}{I \text{ time \%}} \right) \\
&= \ \left( \frac{0.25}{0.25} \right) \ : \ \left( \frac{1 - 0.25}{0.25} \right) \\
&= \ \ \ 1 \ \ \ : \ \left( \frac{0.75}{0.25} \right) \\
&= \ \ \ 1 \ \ \ : \ \ 3
\end{aligned}
$$

## EXERCISE 2

What is the *I:E* ratio if the inspiratory time ratio is 33% or 0.33?

[Answer: *I:E* = 1 : 2]

**EXAMPLE 3**

When the *I* time and *RR* are known:

What is the *I:E* ratio if the inspiratory time is 1.5 sec and the respiratory rate is 15/min?

$I$ time $= 1.5$ sec

$E$ time $= \dfrac{60}{RR} - I$ time

$\qquad = \dfrac{60}{15} - 1.5$

$\qquad = 4 - 1.5$

$\qquad = 2.5$ sec

$I{:}E = I$ time $: E$ time

$\qquad = 1.5 : 2.5$

$\qquad = \left(\dfrac{1.5}{1.5}\right) : \left(\dfrac{2.5}{1.5}\right)$

$\qquad = 1 : 1.67$

**EXERCISE 3**

What is the *I:E* ratio if the inspiratory time is 0.6 sec and the respiratory rate is 20/min?

[Answer: *I:E* = 1 : 4]

**EXAMPLE 4**

When the minute volume ($\dot{V}_E$) and flow rate are known:

Given: $V_T \quad = 800$ mL (0.8 L)

$\qquad RR \quad = 12$/min

$\qquad$ Flow rate $= 40$ L/min

What is the *I:E* ratio?

$I{:}E$ ratio $=$ (Minute volume) : (Flow rate – Minute volume)

$\qquad = (V_T \times RR) : ($Flow rate $- V_T \times RR)$

$\qquad = (0.8 \times 12) : (40 - 0.8 \times 12)$

$\qquad = 9.6 : (40 - 9.6)$

$\qquad = 9.6 : 30.4$

$\qquad$ [divide both sides of this ratio by 9.6]

$\qquad = 1 : 3.2$

**EXERCISE 4**

Given: $V_T \quad = 1000$ mL (1 L)

$\qquad RR \quad = 10$/min

$\qquad$ Flow rate $= 50$ L/min

What is the *I:E* ratio?

[Answer: *I:E* = 1 : 4]

# Self-Assessment Questions

42a. Calculate the *I:E* ratio if the inspiratory time is 0.4 sec and the expiratory time is 0.6 sec.

(A) 1.5 : 1

(B) 1 : 1

(C) 1 : 1.5

(D) 1 : 2

(E) 1.5 : 3

42b. What is the *I:E* ratio if the inspiratory time is 0.5 sec and the expiratory time is 1.5 sec?

(A) 1 : 1

(B) 1 : 2

(C) 1 : 3

(D) 2 : 1

(E) 3 : 1

42c. Calculate the *I:E* ratio when the inspiratory time is 1.2 sec and the expiratory time is 1.8 sec.

(A) 1 : 1.5

(B) 1 : 2

(C) 1 : 2.5

(D) 1 : 3

(E) 3 : 1

42d. Which of the following sets of inspiratory time (*I* time) and expiratory time (*E* time) does not equal an *I:E* ratio of 1:2?

|  | *I* time (sec) | *E* time (sec) |
|---|---|---|
| (A) | 2.0 | 4.0 |
| (B) | 1.5 | 3.0 |
| (C) | 0.8 | 1.6 |
| (D) | 2.0 | 1.0 |
| (E) | 0.25 | 0.5 |

42e. Calculate the *I:E* ratio when the inspiratory time ratio is 25%.

(A) 1 : 3

(B) 1 : 4

(C) 1 : 5

(D) 4 : 1

(E) 3 : 1

42f. What is the *I:E* ratio if the inspiratory time ratio is 40% or 0.4?

(A) 1 : 1.5

(B) 1 : 2

(C) 1 : 2.5

(D) 1 : 3

(E) 1 : 4

42g. The inspiratory time of a mechanical ventilator is set at 30% of one complete respiratory cycle. The *I:E* ratio is about

(A) 1 : 0.3

(B) 1 : 0.7

(C) 1:1

(D) 1:1.3

(E) 1:2.3

42h. Calculate the *I:E* ratio when the inspiratory time on a ventilator is set at 20% of one complete respiratory cycle.

(A) 1:1

(B) 1:2

(C) 1:3

(D) 1:4

(E) 1:5

42i. Which of the following inspiratory time percent (%) settings would give an *I:E* ratio of 1:3?

(A) 10%

(B) 20%

(C) 25%

(D) 30%

(E) 40%

42j. What is the *I:E* ratio if the inspiratory time is 0.5 sec and the respiratory rate is 30/min?

(A) 1:3

(B) 1:4

(C) 1:5

(D) 4:1

(E) 3:1

42k. Calculate the *I:E* ratio for the following settings: inspiratory time = 1 sec, respiratory rate = 20/min.

(A) 1:1

(B) 1:2

(C) 1:3

(D) 1:4

(E) 1:5

42l. Given: inspiratory time = 1.5 sec, respiratory rate = 16/min. Find the expiratory time. What is the *I:E* ratio at these settings?

(A) 0.75 sec; 1:0.5

(B) 1.5 sec; 1:1

(C) 2.25 sec; 1:1.5

(D) 2.63 sec; 1:1.75

(E) 3 sec; 1:2

42m. A patient on a ventilator has an inspiratory time of 1.2 sec and a machine rate of 25/min. What are the expiratory time and *I:E* ratio at these settings?

(A) 0.96 sec; 1:0.8

(B) 1.2 sec; 1:1

(C) 1.44 sec; 1:1.2

(D) 1.68 sec; 1:1.4

(E) 2.16 sec; 1:1.8

42n. Which of the following settings would *not* provide an *I:E* ratio of about 1:0.5?

|     | *I* time (sec) | *RR* |
| --- | --- | --- |
| (A) | 2.0 | 20 |
| (B) | 1.6 | 25 |
| (C) | 1.33 | 30 |
| (D) | 3 | 15 |
| (E) | 1.0 | 40 |

42o. Given: $V_T$ = 1000 mL (1 L), *RR* = 10/min, flow rate = 40 L/min. What is the *I:E* ratio?

(A) 1:3

(B) 1:4

(C) 1:5

(D) 4:1

(E) 3:1

42p. Given: $V_T$ = 1000 mL (1 L), *RR* = 12/min, flow rate = 50 L/min. What is the calculated *I:E* ratio?

(A) 1:3.2

(B) 1:2.8

(C) 1:2.4

(D) 1:2

(E) 1:1.6

42q. Which of the following settings would provide a calculated *I:E* ratio of 1:4?

|     | $V_T$ (mL) | *RR* | Flow rate |
| --- | --- | --- | --- |
| (A) | 800 | 15 | 40 |
| (B) | 800 | 15 | 45 |
| (C) | 800 | 15 | 50 |
| (D) | 800 | 15 | 55 |
| (E) | 800 | 15 | 60 |

42r. A patient on the ventilator has a tidal volume of 850 mL (0.85 L), respiratory rate of 16/min, and flow rate of 50 L/min. Based on these settings, what is the *I:E* ratio? If the flow rate is increased to 60 L/min, will the *E* ratio be longer or shorter?

(A) 1:2.7; *E* ratio will be longer (3.4)

(B) 1:2.7; *E* ratio will be shorter (2.0)

(C) 1:2.4; *E* ratio will be shorter (1.7)

(D) 1:2.1; *E* ratio will be shorter (1.4)

(E) 1:2.1; *E* ratio will be longer (2.8)

42s. A patient has the following settings on a mechanical ventilator: $V_T$ = 750 mL (0.75 L), *RR* = 16/min, flow rate = 50 L/min. Calculate the *I:E* ratio based on these settings. If a *longer E* ratio is desired, should the flow rate be increased or decreased?

(A) 1:1.6; flow rate should be increased

(B) 1:2.4; flow rate should be increased

(C) 1:2.4; flow rate should be decreased

(D) 1:3.2; flow rate should be increased

(E) 1:3.2; flow rate should be decreased

42t. The following settings are found on a mechanical ventilator: $V_T$ = 900 mL (0.9 L), $RR$ = 14/min, flow rate = 55 L/min. What is the calculated *I:E* ratio based on these settings? If a *shorter E* ratio is desired, what should be done to the flow rate?

(A) 1 : 2.9; flow rate should be increased

(B) 1 : 3.1; flow rate should be increased

(C) 1 : 3.1; flow rate should be decreased

(D) 1 : 3.4; flow rate should be increased

(E) 1 : 3.4; flow rate should be decreased

42u. An *I:E* ratio of 1.5:1 is the same as

(A) 1 : 0.5

(B) 1 : 0.67

(C) 1 : 0.8

(D) 1 : 1.5

(E) 1 : 2.5

# CHAPTER

# *43*
# Law of LaPlace

**NOTE**

This equation illustrates two important concepts in respiratory care—one physiological and the other pathophysiological.

## EQUATION

$$P = \frac{2ST}{r}$$

$P$  :  Pressure in dynes/cm$^2$

$ST$  :  Surface tension in dyne/cm

$r$  :  Radius in cm

*Physiological consideration*

In the normal human lungs there are millions of alveoli varying in size. If the surface tensions in these alveoli were exactly alike, the smaller alveoli would empty into the larger alveoli [since low radius ($r$) means a high pressure ($P$) at constant surface tension ($ST$)]. In reality, as the normal alveoli decrease in size, the *relative* amount of surfactant increases, thus lowering the surface tension to maintain an equilibrium in pressure gradient and stability of alveoli of varying sizes.

*Pathophysiological consideration*

The equation shows that the work of breathing ($P$) is directly related to the surface tension ($ST$) of the alveoli. Surfactant deficiency (as in premature lungs and ARDS) causes an increase in pulmonary surface tension, which in turn leads to an increase in the work of breathing. Atelectasis resulting from surfactant deficiency further hinders ventilation because of the inverse relationship between the size of the alveoli ($r$) and work of breathing ($P$).

Artificial and natural surfactants have been used successfully to reduce the surface tension of noncompliant lungs and to improve ventilation in premature infants.

## REFERENCE

Scanlan

## Self-Assessment Questions

43a. In pulmonary physiology, _____ can be used to describe the relationship between work of breathing, surface tension, and size of alveoli.

(A) Law of LaPlace

(B) Dalton's law

(C) Henry's law

(D) Hooke's law

(E) Poiseuille's law

43b. If $P$ in the Law of LaPlace represents work of breathing, it is directly related to the _____ and inversely related to the _____.

(A) radius; surface tension

(B) surface tension; radius

(C) radius; partial pressure of gas

(D) surface tension; partial pressure of gas

(E) tidal volume; respiratory rate

43c. Based on the Law of LaPlace, alveolar units that become _____ cause _____ in the work of breathing.

(A) larger; an increase

(B) smaller; an increase

(C) smaller; a decrease

(D) smaller; no change

(E) larger; no change

43d. Surfactant replacement therapy is effective in _____ the pulmonary surface tension and in _____ the work of breathing.

(A) increasing; decreasing

(B) increasing; increasing

(C) reducing; decreasing

(D) reducing; increasing

(E) stabilizing; increasing

CHAPTER

# *44*
# Lung Volumes and Capacities

NOTES

There are four lung volumes and four lung capacities. Lung volumes are distinct measurements that do not overlap each other. Lung capacities are measurements containing two or more lung volumes (Fig. 31).

Residual volume, functional residual capacity, and total lung capacity cannot be measured directly. They must be measured by an indirect method such as helium dilution, nitrogen washout, body plethysmograph, or radiologic estimation.

Changes in lung volumes/capacities may be used to distinguish restrictive and obstructive lung diseases. In general, restrictive lung diseases show decreases in lung volumes and capacities, whereas obstructive lung diseases have increases in residual volume. Functional residual capacity and total lung capacity may be increased in air trapping or hyperinflation of the lungs because residual volume is part of these two lung capacities (Fig. 32).

## EQUATION 1

$$TLC = IRV + V_T + ERV + RV$$
$$TLC = VC + RV$$
$$TLC = IC + FRC$$

## EQUATION 2

$$VC = IRV + V_T + ERV$$
$$VC = IC + ERV$$
$$VC = TLC - RV$$

## EQUATION 3

$$IC = IRV + V_T$$
$$IC = TLC - FRC$$
$$IC = VC - ERV$$

## EQUATION 4

$$FRC = ERV + RV$$
$$FRC = TLC - IC$$

| | | |
|---|---|---|
| $TLC$ | : | Total lung capacity |
| $VC$ | : | Vital capacity |
| $IC$ | : | Inspiratory capacity |
| $FRC$ | : | Functional residual capacity |
| $IRV$ | : | Inspiratory reserve volume |
| $V_T$ | : | Tidal volume |
| $ERV$ | : | Expiratory reserve volume |
| $RV$ | : | Residual volume |

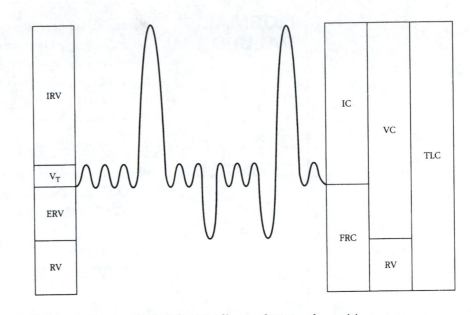

**Figure 31** *Spirogram showing the distribution of lung volumes and capacities.*

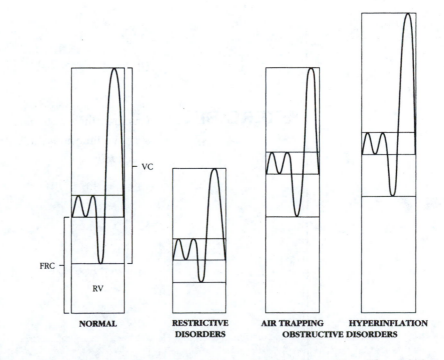

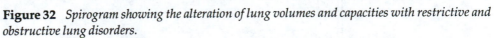

**Figure 32** *Spirogram showing the alteration of lung volumes and capacities with restrictive and obstructive lung disorders.*

## NORMAL VALUES

Normal values depend on a person's gender, age, ethnic origin, height, weight, and smoking history. The traditional normal values for a young adult male are listed below to show calculation of lung volumes and capacities.

$TLC = 6000$ mL; $VC = 4800$ mL; $IC = 3600$ mL; $FRC = 2400$ mL; $IRV = 3100$ mL; $V_T = 500$ mL; $ERV = 1200$ mL; $RV = 1200$ mL

## EXAMPLE 1

What is the calculated residual volume if the total lung capacity is 5800 mL and the vital capacity is 4950 mL?

Since $TLC = VC + RV$ (equation 1),

$$
\begin{aligned}
RV &= TLC - VC \\
&= 5800 - 4950 \\
&= 850 \text{ mL}
\end{aligned}
$$

## EXAMPLE 2

Given: Total lung capacity      $= 6400$ mL
Functional residual capacity   $= 2600$ mL
What is the calculated inspiratory capacity?

$$
\begin{aligned}
IC &= TLC - FRC \text{ (equation 3)}, \\
&= 6400 - 2600 \\
&= 3800 \text{ mL}
\end{aligned}
$$

## EXERCISE 1

If the inspiratory capacity is 3900 mL and the tidal volume is 620 mL, what is the calculated inspiratory reserve volume?

[Answer: $IRV = 3280$ mL]

## EXERCISE 2

Calculate the functional residual capacity if the expiratory reserve volume and residual volume are 1100 mL and 1500 mL, respectively.

[Answer: $FRC = 2600$ mL]

**EXERCISE 3**    What is the calculated tidal volume if the inspiratory capacity is 3450 mL and the inspiratory reserve volume is 2950 mL?

[Answer: $V_T = 500$ mL]

**REFERENCES**    Madama; Ruppel

**SEE**    *Appendix J, Normal Values for Lung Volumes, Capacities, and Ventilation.*

## Self-Assessment Questions

44a.  The sum of *IRV* and $V_T$ is equal to

  (A) *VC*

  (B) *TLC*

  (C) *IC*

  (D) *FRC*

  (E) *ERV*

44b.  A patient's vital capacity can be calculated by the equation

  (A) $VC = IRV + ERV$

  (B) $VC = TLC - IRV$

  (C) $VC = IRV + V_T$

  (D) $VC = TLC - RV$

  (E) $VC = FRC - RV$

44c.  Which of the following cannot be measured by simple spirometry?

  (A) *VC*

  (B) $V_T$

  (C) *IRV*

  (D) *ERV*

  (E) *RV*

44d.  A patient's vital capacity can be calculated by using which of the following equations?

  I.    $TLC - RV = VC$

  II.   $IC + FRC = VC$

  III.  $IRV + V_T + ERV = VC$

  IV.   $FRC + V_T = VC$

  V.    $IC + ERV = VC$

  (A) I and II only

(B) II and IV only

(C) III and V only

(D) I, II and IV only

(E) I, III, and V only

44e. Which of the following equations is incorrect for calculating the total lung capacity (TLC)?

(A) $TLC = IRV + V_T + ERV + RV$

(B) $TLC = VC + RV$

(C) $TLC = IC + FRC$

(D) $TLC = IRV + V_T + ERV$

(E) $TLC = IC + ERV + RV$

44f. Which of the following equations is incorrect for calculating the vital capacity (VC)?

(A) $VC = IRV + V_T$

(B) $VC = IRV + V_T + ERV$

(C) $VC = IC + ERV$

(D) $VC = IC + FRC - RV$

(E) $VC = TLC - RV$

44g. All of the following equations are correct with the *exception* of

(A) $IC = IRV + V_T$

(B) $V_T = IC - IRV$

(C) $FRC = ERV + RV$

(D) $ERV = VC - IC$

(E) $VC = IC + FRC$

*MATCHING:* Match the lung capacities with the values listed in Column II. Use only four answers from Column II.

Given: $IRV = 3100$ mL, $V_T = 500$ mL, $ERV = 1200$ mL, $RV = 1200$ mL.

| Column I | | Column II | |
|---|---|---|---|
| 44h. | VC | (A) | 6000 mL |
| 44i. | FRC | (B) | 4800 mL |
| 44j. | IC | (C) | 3600 mL |
| 44k. | TLC | (D) | 2400 mL |
| | | (E) | 1700 mL |

44l. A pulmonary function study shows the following: $IRV = 1200$ mL, $V_T = 500$ mL, $ERV = 1000$ mL. Based on these values, the patient's TLC would be

(A) 1700 mL

(B) 1700 mL plus RV

(C) 2700 mL

(D) 2700 mL minus RV

(E) 2700 mL plus RV

44m. Studies on a patient reveal the following: $IRV = 1600$ mL, $V_T = 500$ mL, $ERV = 1000$ mL. On the basis of these data, the patient's TLC would be

(A) 2100 mL minus RV

(B) 2600 mL plus RV

(C) 3100 mL

(D) 3100 mL minus *RV*

(E) 3100 mL plus *RV*

For questions 44n–44q, use the following lung volumes to calculate the lung capacities for the next four questions:

$IRV = 3000$ mL, $V_T = 650$ mL, $ERV = 1100$ mL, $RV = 1150$ mL

**44n.** Total lung capacity (*TLC*) is

(A) 2900 mL

(B) 3650 mL

(C) 4800 mL

(D) 5900 mL

(E) none of the above

**44o.** Vital capacity (*VC*) is

(A) 2250 mL

(B) 2900 mL

(C) 3650 mL

(D) 4750 mL

(E) 5900 mL

**44p.** Inspiratory capacity (*IC*) is

(A) 2250 mL

(B) 2900 mL

(C) 3650 mL

(D) 4750 mL

(E) 5900 mL

**44q.** Functional residual capacity (*FRC*) is

(A) 2250 mL

(B) 2900 mL

(C) 3650 mL

(D) 4750 mL

(E) 5900 mL

**44r.** Calculate the residual volume when the total lung capacity is 6200 mL and the vital capacity is 4900 mL.

(A) 1100 mL

(B) 1200 mL

(C) 1300 mL

(D) 1400 mL

(E) 11.1 L

**44s.** Given: total lung capacity = 5500 mL, functional residual capacity = 2300 mL. What is the inspiratory capacity (*IC*)?

(A) 2300 mL

(B) 3200 mL

(C) 5500 mL

(D) 7800 mL

(E) residual volume required to calculate *IC*

44t.   If the inspiratory capacity is 3200 mL and the tidal volume is 500 mL, what is the inspiratory reserve volume (*IRV*)?

(A) 500 mL

(B) 2700 mL

(C) 3200 mL

(D) 3700 mL

(E)  vital capacity required to calculate *IRV*

## CHAPTER

# *45*
# Mean Airway Pressure (*MAWP*)

**NOTES**

The mean airway pressure (*MAWP*) is the average pressure in the airways over a series of breathing cycles, usually measured during mechanical ventilation.

*MAWP* is increased when there is an increase in any of the following: peak inspiratory pressure, respiratory rate, inspiratory time. *MAWP* is also increased when expiratory retard (hold), pressure support, or PEEP is used.

An increase in *MAWP* causes the cardiac output to fall, particularly in patients with unstable hemodynamic status. Therefore, *MAWP* should be kept at the lowest possible level by limiting the factors listed above, particularly the *I* time and PEEP.

## EQUATION

$$MAWP = \left[\frac{RR \times I\,\text{time}}{60}\right] \times (PIP - PEEP) + PEEP$$

| | | |
|---|---|---|
| *MAWP* | : | Mean airway pressure in cm $H_2O$ |
| *RR* | : | Respiratory rate / min |
| *I* time | : | Inspiratory time in sec |
| *PIP* | : | Peak inspiratory pressure in cm $H_2O$ |
| PEEP | : | Positive end-expiratory pressure in cm $H_2O$ |

## NORMAL VALUE

Use serial measurements to establish trend.

## EXAMPLE 1

When PEEP is used:

Given: *RR*   = 45 / min
      *I* time   = 0.5 sec
      *PIP*   = 35 cm $H_2O$
      PEEP   = 5 cm $H_2O$

Calculate the mean airway pressure.

$$
\begin{aligned}
MAWP &= \left[\frac{RR \times I\,\text{time}}{60}\right] \times (PIP - PEEP) + PEEP \\
&= \left[\frac{45 \times 0.5}{60}\right] \times (35 - 5) + 5 \\
&= \left[\frac{22.5}{60}\right] \times 30 + 5 \\
&= [0.375] \times 30 + 5 \\
&= 11.25 + 5 \\
&= 16.25 \text{ or } 16 \text{ cm } H_2O
\end{aligned}
$$

## EXAMPLE 2

When PEEP is not used (assuming same *PIP*):

Given: *RR*   = 45 / min
      *I* time   = 0.5 sec
      *PIP*   = 35 cm $H_2O$
      PEEP   = 0 cm $H_2O$

Calculate the mean airway pressure.

$$MAWP = \left[ \frac{RR \times I\text{ time}}{60} \right] \times (PIP - PEEP) + PEEP$$

$$= \left[ \frac{45 \times 0.5}{60} \right] \times (35 - 0) + 0$$

$$= \left[ \frac{22.5}{60} \right] \times 35 + 0$$

$$= [0.375] \times 35 + 0$$

$$= 13.13 + 0$$

$$= 13.13 \text{ or } 13 \text{ cm } H_2O$$

## EXERCISE 1

When PEEP is used:

Given: $RR$    =   16/min

       $I$ time   =   1 sec

       $PIP$     =   40 cm $H_2O$

       PEEP   =   10 cm $H_2O$

What is the calculated mean airway pressure?

[Answer: $MAWP$ = 18 cm $H_2O$]

## EXERCISE 2

When PEEP is not used (assuming same PIP):

Given: $RR$    =   16/min

       $I$ time   =   1 sec

       $PIP$     =   40 cm $H_2O$

       PEEP   =   0 cm $H_2O$

Calculate the mean airway pressure.

[Answer: $MAWP$ = 10.67 or 11 cm $H_2O$]

## REFERENCES

Burton; Moser

## Self-Assessment Questions

45a.  Given: $RR$ = 20/min, $I$ time = 0.5 sec, peak inspiratory pressure = 40 cm $H_2O$, PEEP = 5 cm $H_2O$. Calculate the mean airway pressure (*MAWP*).

(A) 11 cm $H_2O$

(B) 13 cm $H_2O$

(C) 15 cm $H_2O$

(D) 17 cm $H_2O$

(E) 19 cm $H_2O$

45b.  Given: $RR$ = 26/min, $I$ time = 1.0 sec, PIP = 65 cm $H_2O$, PEEP = 15 cm $H_2O$. Calculate the mean airway pressure (*MAWP*).

(A) 21.7 cm $H_2O$

(B) 30.3 cm $H_2O$

(C) 36.7 cm $H_2O$

(D) 39.4 cm $H_2O$

(E) 42.1 cm $H_2O$

45c.  A patient has the following settings on a mechanical ventilator: $RR$ = 16/min, $I$ time = 1.5 sec, PIP = 50 cm $H_2O$, PEEP = 0 cm $H_2O$. What is the calculated mean airway pressure (*MAWP*)?

(A) 16 cm $H_2O$

(B) 20 cm $H_2O$

(C) 24 cm $H_2O$

(D) 30 cm $H_2O$

(E) 32 cm $H_2O$

45d.  Positive end-expiratory pressure (PEEP) of 10 cm $H_2O$ is added to the patient in the preceding question. The new parameters are as follows: $RR$ = 16/min, $I$ time = 1.5 sec, PIP = 55 cm $H_2O$, PEEP = 10 cm $H_2O$. What is the calculated mean airway pressure (*MAWP*)?

(A) 16 cm $H_2O$

(B) 18 cm $H_2O$

(C) 23 cm $H_2O$

(D) 28 cm $H_2O$

(E) 30 cm $H_2O$

45e.  A neonate is being ventilated by a pressure-limited ventilator with these settings: $RR$ = 36/min, $I$ time = 0.5 sec, PIP = 35 cm $H_2O$, PEEP = 5 cm $H_2O$. Based on this information, calculate the mean airway pressure (*MAWP*).

(A) 9 cm $H_2O$

(B) 14 cm $H_2O$

(C) 20 cm $H_2O$

(D) 30 cm $H_2O$

(E) 40 cm $H_2O$

45f.  An infant ventilator has these settings: $RR$ = 30/min, $I$ time = 0.5 sec, PIP = 25 cm $H_2O$, PEEP = 6 cm $H_2O$. What is the approximate mean airway pressure (*MAWP*)? If the $I$ time is increased to 0.6 sec, would the *MAWP* be higher or lower if other parameters remain unchanged?

(A) 9 cm $H_2O$; higher (10 cm $H_2O$)

    (B) 11 cm $H_2O$; lower (10 cm $H_2O$)

    (C) 11 cm $H_2O$; higher (12 cm $H_2O$)

    (D) 17 cm $H_2O$; higher (18 cm $H_2O$)

    (E) 17 cm $H_2O$; lower (16 cm $H_2O$)

45g. A recent ventilator check in the NICU revealed the following ventilator settings: $RR$ = 40/min, $I$ time = 0.4 sec, PIP = 30 cm $H_2O$, PEEP = 0 cm $H_2O$. What is the neonate's approximate mean airway pressure (*MAWP*)? If PEEP of 5 cm $H_2O$ is added to the ventilator settings, what will be the new *MAWP* if other parameters remain unchanged?

    (A) 7 cm $H_2O$; 12 cm $H_2O$

    (B) 7 cm $H_2O$; 13 cm $H_2O$

    (C) 8 cm $H_2O$; 12 cm $H_2O$

    (D) 8 cm $H_2O$; 13 cm $H_2O$

    (E) 10 cm $H_2O$; 15 cm $H_2O$

# CHAPTER

# *46*

# Mean Arterial Pressure (*MAP*)

## EQUATION

$$MAP = \frac{BP_{\text{systolic}} + 2\,BP_{\text{diastolic}}}{3}$$

| | | |
|---|---|---|
| *MAP* | : | Mean arterial pressure in mm Hg |
| $BP_{\text{systolic}}$ | : | Systolic blood pressure in mm Hg |
| $BP_{\text{diastolic}}$ | : | Diastolic blood pressure in mm Hg |

### NOTES

This equation calculates the mean (average) arterial blood pressure in the systemic circulation. A normal value of 60 mm Hg is considered the minimum *MAP* needed to maintain adequate tissue perfusion.

*MAP* is directly related to the systemic vascular resistance (*SVR*) and the cardiac output (*CO*):

$$MAP = SVR \times CO$$

In patients whose systemic vascular resistance is low (e.g., loss of venous tone) or whose cardiac output is low (e.g., CHF), the *MAP* will be low. The *MAP* is usually high in patients with systemic hypertension.

This equation uses $2 \times BP_{\text{diastolic}}$ because the diastolic phase is assumed to be twice as long as the systolic phase. When the heart rate is greater than 120/min, this equation loses its accuracy.

## NORMAL VALUE

>60 mm Hg

## EXAMPLE

Given: $BP_{\text{systolic}}$ = 120 mm Hg
$\quad\quad\quad BP_{\text{diastolic}}$ = 80 mm Hg

Calculate the mean arterial pressure.

$$
\begin{aligned}
MAP &= \frac{BP_{\text{systolic}} + 2\,BP_{\text{diastolic}}}{3} \\[6pt]
&= \frac{120 + 2 \times 80}{3} \\[6pt]
&= \frac{120 + 160}{3} \\[6pt]
&= \frac{280}{3} \\[6pt]
&= 93 \text{ mm Hg}
\end{aligned}
$$

## EXERCISE

Given: Systolic blood pressure = 110 mm Hg
$\quad\quad\quad$ Diastolic blood pressure = 50 mm Hg

Calculate the *MAP*.

[Answer: *MAP* = 70 mm Hg]

**REFERENCE**   Bustin

**SEE**   *Vascular Resistance: Systemic (SVR); Cardiac Output (CO): Fick's Estimated Method.*

## Self-Assessment Questions

46a.  Given: systolic blood pressure = 100 mm Hg, diastolic blood pressure = 60 mm Hg. Calculate the mean arterial pressure (*MAP*).

(A)  60 mm Hg

(B)  73 mm Hg

(C)  80 mm Hg

(D)  100 mm Hg

(E)  160 mm Hg

46b.  Given: systolic blood pressure = 110 mm Hg, diastolic blood pressure = 70 mm Hg. Calculate the mean arterial pressure (*MAP*).

(A)  35 mm Hg

(B)  60 mm Hg

(C)  70 mm Hg

(D)  83 mm Hg

(E)  90 mm Hg

46c.  A patient has a systemic blood pressure reading of 90/60 mm Hg. The calculated mean arterial pressure (*MAP*) is therefore

(A)  50 mm Hg

(B)  60 mm Hg

(C)  70 mm Hg

(D)  75 mm Hg

(E)  90 mm Hg

CHAPTER

# 47
# Metric Conversion: Length

## CONVERSION TABLE

| Millimeters | Centimeters | Inches | Feet | Yards | Meters |
|---|---|---|---|---|---|
| 1 | 0.1 | 0.03937 | 0.00328 | 0.00109 | 0.001 |
| 10.0 | 1 | 0.3937 | 0.03281 | 0.0109 | 0.01 |
| 25.4 | 2.54 | 1 | 0.0833 | 0.0278 | 0.0254 |
| 304.8 | 30.48 | 12.0 | 1 | 0.3333 | 0.3048 |
| 914.40 | 91.44 | 36.0 | 3.0 | 1 | 0.9144 |
| 1000.0 | 100.0 | 39.37 | 3.2808 | 1.0936 | 1 |

**EXAMPLE 1**   Convert 8 inches (in.) to millimeters (mm).

Step 1. From the conversion table, 1 in. = 25.4 mm.

Step 2. 8 in. = $(8 \times 25.4)$ mm or 203.2 mm

**EXAMPLE 2**   Convert 40 centimeters (cm) to feet (ft).

Step 1. From the conversion table, 1 cm = 0.03281 ft.

Step 2. 40 cm = $(40 \times 0.03281)$ ft or 1.3124 ft

**EXAMPLE 3**   Mr. James is 5'8" tall. What is the centimeter (cm) equivalent?

Step 1. From the conversion table, 1 ft = 12 in.

Step 2. 5 ft = $(5 \times 12)$ in. = 60 in.

Step 3. 5 ft 8 in. is therefore 68 in. $(60 + 8)$.

Step 4. From the conversion table, 1 in. = 2.54 cm.

Step 5. 68 in. = $(68 \times 2.54)$ cm or 172.72 cm.

**EXAMPLE 4**   Ms. Malby is 160 cm tall. How tall is she in feet and inches?

Step 1. From the conversion table, 1 cm = 0.3937 in.

Step 2. 160 cm = $(160 \times 0.3937)$ in. = 63 in.

Step 3. From the conversion table, 1 ft = 12 in.

Step 4. 63 in. = $(63 / 12)$ ft = 5.25 ft or 5 ft 3 in.

*NOTES*

If a calculator is used to obtain the answer, the number in front of the decimal point represents the feet; the number after the decimal point should be multiplied by 12 to obtain the remaining height in inches. In Example 4, 63/12 = 5.25, the number in front of the decimal point (5) is the height in feet. The number after the decimal point (0.25) is multiplied by 12 for the remaining height in inches: 0.25 × 12 = 3 inches. The height is therefore 5'3".

## EXERCISE 1

A patient tells you that her height is 5'5". If you need to enter her height in the pulmonary function data sheet in centimeters (cm), what should it be?

[Answer: Height in cm = 165.1 or 165 cm]

## EXERCISE 2

Mr. Hall is 176 cm tall. Convert his height to feet and inches.

[Answer: Height in ft and in. = 5'9".]

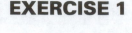

## Self-Assessment Questions

47a. Convert 280 millimeters (mm) to inches (in.)

(A) 1.02 in.

(B) 11.02 in.

(C) 110.2 in.

(D) 7112 in.

47b. Convert 46 meters (m) to feet (ft).

(A) 14 ft

(B) 15.1 ft

(C) 140 ft

(D) 151 ft

47c. Convert 12 inches (in.) to centimeters (cm).

(A) 0.30 cm

(B) 3.05 cm

(C) 30.48 cm

(D) 304.8 cm

47d. Convert 1.6 feet (ft) to millimeters (mm).

(A) 487.7 mm

(B) 4877 mm

(C) 521.4 mm

(D) 5214 mm

47e. A patient, Ms. Smith, is 5'6" tall. What is the centimeter (cm) equivalent?

(A) 154.10 cm

(B) 1541 cm

(C) 167.6 cm

(D) 1676 cm

47f. Mr. Jackson is 180 cm tall. Convert this height to feet and inches.

(A) 5 ft 8 in.

(B) 5 ft 9 in.

(C) 5 ft 10 in.

(D) 5 ft 11 in.

47g. A patient is 5'9" tall. If you need to record the height in centimeters (cm), what should it be?

(A) 167 cm

(B) 175 cm

(C) 179 cm

(D) 182 cm

47h. Mr. Hall runs 1600 meters every morning. This is the same as how many feet?

(A) 524 ft

(B) 4800 ft

(C) 5249 ft

(D) 48000 ft

CHAPTER

# *48*
# Metric Conversion: Volume

## CONVERSION TABLE

| Milliliters | Microliters | Liters | Fluid Ounces | Pints | Quarts |
|---|---|---|---|---|---|
| 1 | 1000 | 0.001 | 0.03381 | 0.00211 | 0.001055 |
| 0.001 | 1 | 0.000001 | 0.0000338 | 0.00000211 | 0.000001055 |
| 1000 | 1000000 | 1 | 33.8 | 2.11 | 1.55 |
| 29.57 | 29570 | 0.02957 | 1 | 0.0625 | 0.0315 |
| 473.16 | 47316 | 0.47316 | 16.0 | 1 | 0.5 |
| 946.32 | 94632 | 0.94632 | 32.0 | 2.0 | 1 |

### EXAMPLE 1

Convert 12 fluid ounces (fl oz) to milliliters (mL).

Step 1. From the conversion table, 1 fl oz = 29.57 mL.

Step 2. 12 fl oz = $(12 \times 29.57)$ mL or 354.84 mL.

### EXAMPLE 2

Convert 2 liters (L) to pints (pt).

Step 1. From the conversion table, 1 L = 2.11 pt.

Step 2. 2 L = $(2 \times 2.11)$ pt or 4.22 pt.

### EXAMPLE 3

A blood gas analyzer has the capability to analyze blood samples as low as 100 microliters (μL). What is the milliliter (mL) equivalent?

Step 1. From the conversion table, 1 μL = 0.001 mL.

Step 2. 100 μL = $(100 \times 0.001)$ mL = 0.1 mL.

### EXAMPLE 4

A large-volume aerosol unit holds 1000 ml of sterile water. Convert this volume to fluid ounces (fl oz).

Step 1. From the conversion table, 1 mL = 0.03381 fl oz.

Step 2. 1000 mL = $(1000 \times 0.03381)$ fl oz = 33.81 fl oz

**EXERCISE 1**

In order to analyze a capillary blood gas sample, a minimum sample size of 60 microliters (μL) is needed. What is the milliliter (mL) equivalent?

[Answer: Sample size in mL = 0.06 mL]

**EXERCISE 2**

Before using a concentrated disinfectant solution, 2 liters of water must be added. How much water in fluid ounces (fl oz) should be added to prepare this disinfectant solution before use?

[Answer: Water to be added = 67.6 fl oz]

## Self-Assessment Questions

48a. Convert 32 fluid ounces (fl oz) to milliliters (mL).

(A) 1.08 mL

(B) 94.6 mL

(C) 946 mL

(D) 1008 mL

48b. Convert 6 pints (pt) to liters.

(A) 2.12 L

(B) 2.84 L

(C) 21.2 L

(D) 28.4 L

48c. Convert 2 liters (L) to milliliters (mL).

(A) 20 mL

(B) 200 mL

(C) 2000 mL

(D) 20000 mL

48d. Convert 300 microliters (μL) to milliliters (mL).

(A) 0.003 mL

(B) 0.03 mL

(C) 0.3 mL

(D) 3 mL

48e. A blood gas syringe contains 0.4 mL of arterial blood sample. What is the microliters (μL) equivalent?

(A) 0.4 μL

(B) 4 μL

(C) 40 μL

(D) 400 μL

48f. A heated cascade holds 1.6 quarters of sterile water. Convert this volume to liters (L).

(A) 1.51 L

(B) 1.78 L

(C) 15.1 L

(D) 17.8 L

48g. The minimum sample size for a blood gas analyzer is 80 microliters (μL). What is the milliliter (mL) equivalent?

(A) 0.008 mL

(B) 0.08 mL

(C) 0.8 mL

(D) 8 mL

48h. A concentrated cleaning solution is being diluted with 12 quarts of water before use. How much water in fluid ounces (fl oz) should be added?

(A) 36.5 fl oz

(B) 365 fl oz

(C) 38.4 fl oz

(D) 384 fl oz

# CHAPTER

# *49*

# Metric Conversion: Weight

## CONVERSION TABLE

| Milligrams | Grams | Kilograms | Ounces | Pounds |
|---|---|---|---|---|
| 1 | 0.001 | 0.000001 | 0.0000352 | 0.0000022 |
| 1000 | 1 | 0.001 | 0.0352 | 0.0022 |
| 1000000 | 1000 | 1 | 35.2 | 2.2 |
| 28410 | 28.41 | 0.02841 | 1 | 0.0625 |
| 454545 | 454.545 | 0.4545 | 16.0 | 1 |

**EXAMPLE 1**   Convert 78 kilograms (kg) to pounds (lb).

Step 1. From the conversion table, 1 kg = 2.2 lb.

Step 2. 78 kg = (78 × 2.2) lb or 171.6 lb.

**EXAMPLE 2**   Convert 120 pounds (lb) to kilograms (kg).

Step 1. From the conversion table, 1 lb = 0.4545 kg.

Step 2. 120 lb = (120 × 0.4545) or 54.54 kg.

**EXAMPLE 3**   Convert 6 lb 7 oz to grams (gm) and kilograms (kg).

Step 1. From the conversion table, 1 lb = 16 oz.

Step 2. 6 lb = (6 × 16) oz = 96 oz.

Step 3. 6 lb 7 oz = (96 + 7) oz = 103 oz.

Step 4. From the conversion table, 1 oz = 28.41 gm.

Step 5. 103 oz = (103 × 28.41) gm = 2926.23 gm.

Step 6. From the conversion table, 1 gm = 0.001 kg.

Step 7. 2926.23 gm = (2926.23 × 0.001) = 2.92623 or 2.93 kg.

6 lb 7 oz = 2926.23 gm or 2.93 kg.

**EXAMPLE 4**   A premature infant weights 800 grams (g) at birth. What is this birth weight in pounds (lb) and ounces (oz)?

Step 1. From the conversion table, 1 g = 0.0022 lb.

Step 2. 800 g = (800 × 0.0022) lb = 1.76 lb or 1 lb 12 oz.

800 gm = 1 lb 12 oz.

*NOTES*

In step 2 of example 4, the number in front of the decimal point represents the weight in lb; the number after the decimal point should be multiplied by 16 to obtain the remaining weight in oz. In this example, 1 (the number in front of the decimal point) is the weight in lb; 0.76 (the number after the decimal point) is multiplied by 16 for the remaining weight in oz: 0.76 × 16 = 12.16 oz or 12 oz. The birth weight is therefore 1 lb 12 oz.

**EXERCISE 1**    Mr. Dade, who weighs 150 lbs, is ready for the pulmonary function study. What is his weight in kilograms (kg)?

[Answer: Weight = 68.18 kg]

**EXERCISE 2**    The birth weight of a neonate is 3 lb 12 oz. What is this birth weight in grams (gm) and kilograms (kg)?

[Answer: Birth weight = 1704.6 gm or 1.7 kg]

## Self-Assessment Questions

49a.  Convert 1200 grams (g) to pounds (lb).

(A) 0.26 lb

(B) 0.32 lb

(C) 2.64 lb

(D) 3.18 lb

49b.  Convert 150 pounds (lb) to kilograms (kg).

(A) 59.22 kg

(B) 62.15 kg

(C) 68.18 kg

(D) 70.02 kg

49c.  Convert 77 kilograms (kg) to pounds (lb).

(A) 169.4 lb

(B) 172.9 lb

(C) 174.2 lb

(D) 177.7 lb

49d.  Convert 8 lb 4 oz to grams (gm).

(A) 3675 gm

(B) 3700 gm

(C) 3725 gm

(D) 3750 gm

49e. Convert 8 lb 7 oz to kilograms (kg).

(A) 3.66 kg

(B) 3.84 kg

(C) 4.07 kg

(D) 4.22 kg

49f. A neonate weighs 3500 grams (g) at birth. Record this birth weight in pounds (lb) and ounces (oz).

(A) 7 lb 7 oz

(B) 7 lb 11 oz

(C) 7 lb 14 oz

(D) 8 lb 1 oz

49g. The birth weight of a neonate is 4 lb 6 oz. What is this birth weight in grams (gm) and kilograms (kg)?

(A) 181.8 gm, 18.18 kg

(B) 1818 gm, 1.818 kg

(C) 198.8 gm, 1.988 kg

(D) 1988 gm, 1.988 kg

49h. A concentration of 1 g per 100 mL is the same as _____ mg per 100 mL.

(A) 10

(B) 100

(C) 1000

(D) 10000

49i. An 0.5% bronchodilator solution has a concentration of 0.5 g per 100 mL. This is the same as how many milligrams per 100 mL?

(A) 500 mg

(B) 5000 mg

(C) 50000 mg

(D) 500000 mg

# CHAPTER

# *50*
# Minute Ventilation during IMV

This equation is used to calculate the minute ventilation during intermittent mandatory ventilation (IMV) or similar modes of ventilation.

In some ventilators or special circuits, it is possible to measure the total minute ventilation during IMV. Otherwise, it becomes necessary to use this equation to measure the total minute ventilation. The patient tidal volume and respiratory rate are average measurements over a period of 1 minute.

The ventilator tidal volume ($V_T$ mech) should be the corrected tidal volume.

## EQUATION

$$\dot{V}_E = V_T\,mech \times RR\,mech) + (V_T\,spon \times RR\,spon)$$

$\dot{V}_E$      :    Expired minute ventilation in L/min

$V_T$ mech :    Mechanical ventilator tidal volume in mL

$RR$ mech :    Mechanical ventilator respiratory rate/min

$V_T$ spon :    Patient's spontaneous tidal volume in mL

$RR$ spon :    Patient's spontaneous respiratory rate/min

## EXAMPLE

Given: $V_T$ mech    =    900 mL

        $RR$ mech      =    4/min

        $V_T$ spon      =    250 mL

        $RR$ spon      =    10/min

Calculate the expired minute ventilation ($\dot{V}_E$).

$\dot{V}_E$   =   $(V_T\,mech \times RR\,mech) + (V_T\,spon \times RR\,spon)$

     =   $(900 \times 4) + (250 \times 10)$

     =   $3600 + 2500$

     =   6100 mL/min or 6.1 L/min

## EXERCISE

Given: $V_T$ mech    =    1000 mL

        $RR$ mech      =    6/min

        $V_T$ spon      =    240 mL

        $RR$ spon      =    10/min

Calculate the expired minute ventilation ($\dot{V}_E$).

[Answer: $\dot{V}_E = 8.4$ L/min]

## SEE

*Corrected Tidal Volume ($V_T$).*

## Self-Assessment Questions

50a. Given: $V_T$ mech = 1000 mL, $RR$ mech = 5/min, $V_T$ spon = 200 mL, $RR$ spon = 10/min. Calculate the approximate minute ventilation ($\dot{V}_E$).

(A) 4 L

(B) 5 L

(C) 6 L

(D) 7 L

(E) 8 L

50b. The following average measurements are obtained from a ventilator check while the patient is on the SIMV mode: $V_T$ mech = 900 mL, $RR$ mech = 8/min, $V_T$ spon = 350 mL, $RR$ spon = 10/min. What is the minute ventilation?

(A) 3.5 L

(B) 7.2 L

(C) 8.3 L

(D) 10.7 L

(E) 12.9 L

50c. While on the SIMV mode, a patient was breathing spontaneously at a rate of 12/min and an average tidal volume of 300 mL. If the ventilator tidal volume and rate were set at 850 mL and 4/min, respectively, what is the approximate minute ventilation?

(A) 6 L

(B) 7 L

(C) 8 L

(D) 9 L

(E) 10 L

# *51*
# Minute Ventilation: Expired and Alveolar

## NOTES

These equations are used to calculate the expired minute ventilation and the alveolar minute ventilation.

The expired minute ventilation ($\dot{V}_E$) estimates a patient's ventilation effort (Fig. 33). The alveolar minute ventilation ($\dot{V}_A$) is more meaningful; it accurately reflects the effective ventilation—the portion of ventilation capable of taking part in gas exchange (Fig. 34).

Normally 1 mL/lb body weight is used to estimate the anatomic deadspace. If the physiologic deadspace is significant, the $V_D$ should be measured.

In mechanical ventilation, the $V_T$ should be the corrected tidal volume.

## EQUATION 1

$$\dot{V}_E = V_T \times RR$$

## EQUATION 2

$$\dot{V}_A = (V_T - V_D) \times RR$$

$\dot{V}_E$ : Expired minute ventilation in L/min
$\dot{V}_A$ : Alveolar minute ventilation in L/min
$V_T$ : Tidal volume in mL
$V_D$ : Deadspace volume in mL
$RR$ : Respiratory rate/min

## EXAMPLE

Given: $V_T$ = 600 mL
$\quad\quad V_D$ = 150 mL
$\quad\quad RR$ = 12/min

Calculate the expired minute ventilation ($\dot{V}_E$) and the alveolar minute ventilation ($\dot{V}_A$).

$\dot{V}_E$ = $V_T \times RR$
$\quad$ = $600 \times 12$
$\quad$ = 7200 mL/min or 7.2 L/min

$\dot{V}_A$ = $(V_T - V_D) \times RR$
$\quad$ = $(600 - 150) \times 12$
$\quad$ = $450 \times 12$
$\quad$ = 5400 mL/min or 5.4 L/min

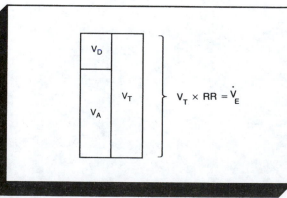

**Figure 33** *Relationship of tidal volume ($V_T$) and expired minute ventilation ($\dot{V}_E$). RR is respiratory rate per minute.*

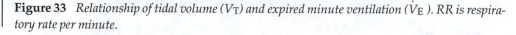

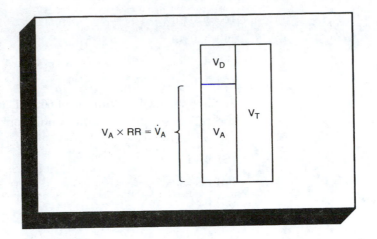

**Figure 34**  *Relationship of alveolar volume ($V_A$) and alveolar minute ventilation ($\dot{V}_A$). RR is respiratory rate per minute.*

**EXERCISE**

Given: $V_T$ = 550 mL

$V_D$ = 100 mL

$RR$ = 12/min

Calculate the $\dot{V}_E$ and the $\dot{V}_A$

[Answer: $\dot{V}_E$ = 6.6 L/min; $\dot{V}_A$ = 5.4 L/min]

**REFERENCE**

Madama

**SEE**

*Deadspace to Tidal Volume Ratio ($V_D/V_T$).*
*Corrected Tidal Volume ($V_T$).*

## Self-Assessment Questions

51a. The anatomic dead space can be estimated to be

(A) 1 mL/kg of body weight

(B) 1 mL/lb of body weight

(C) 10 mL/kg of body weight

(D) 10 mL/lb of body weight

(E) 100 mL

51b. A patient has an expired tidal volume of 600 mL. If the patient weights 120 lb, the estimated alveolar tidal volume is

(A) 600 mL

(B) 520 mL

(C) 480 mL

(D) 420 mL

(E) 120 mL

51c. A patient has a tidal volume of 600 mL and a respiratory rate of 12/min. What is the patient's expired minute ventilation?

(A) 3.8 L

(B) 4.4 L

(C) 5.4 L

(D) 6.8L

(E) 7.2 L

For Questions 51d–51f, given: $V_T = 800$ mL, $V_D = 200$ mL, $RR = 10$/min.

51d. What is the alveolar minute ventilation?

(A) 600 mL

(B) 800 mL

(C) 6 L

(D) 8 L

(E) none of the above

51e. What is the alveolar tidal volume?

(A) 200 mL

(B) 400 mL

(C) 600 mL

(D) 800 mL

(E) none of the above

51f. The calculated $\dot{V}_E$ is

(A) 600 mL

(B) 800 mL

(C) 6 L

(D) 8 L

(E) none of the above

51g. A patient is breathing at a tidal volume of 600 mL and a respiratory rate of 12/min. What is the estimated alveolar minute ventilation if the patient weighs 150 lb?

(A) 3.8 L

(B) 4.4 L

(C) 5.4 L

(D) 6.8 L

(E) 7.2 L

51h. Exhaled volumes are collected from a patient over a 1-min interval; during this time 14 breaths are recorded. If the total expired volume is 10 L, the average tidal volume is about

(A) 140 mL

(B) 714 mL

(C) 1000 mL

(D) 1100 mL

(E) 1400 mL

51i. What is the expected alveolar minute ventilation for a 68-kg (150-lb) patient who has a tidal volume of 500 mL and a respiratory rate of 20/min?

(A) 3 L

(B) 7 L

(C) 8 L

(D) 9 L

(E) 10 L

51j. Given: $V_T$ = 780 mL, $V_D$ = 160 mL, $RR$ = 14/min. Calculate the approximate expired minute ventilation ($\dot{V}_E$) and alveolar minute ventilation ($\dot{V}_A$).

(A) 7.8 L; 6.2 L

(B) 9.4 L; 7.8 L

(C) 10.9 L; 7.8 L

(D) 10.9 L; 8.7 L

(E) 10.9 L; 9.4L

51k. A patient weighing 130 lb has an average $V_T$ of 610 mL and respiratory rate of 16/min. What is the estimated dead space volume ($V_D$)? What is the calculated alveolar minute ventilation ($\dot{V}_A$)?

(A) 100 mL; 6.10 L

(B) 100 mL; 7.68 L

(C) 130 mL; 7.68 L

(D) 130 mL; 9.76 L

(E) 150 mL; 9.76 L

51l. Which of the following measurements provide the best (largest) alveolar minute ventilation?

|  | $V_T$ (mL) | $V_D$ (mL) | $RR$ |
|---|---|---|---|
| (A) | 800 | 110 | 15 |
| (B) | 750 | 130 | 18 |
| (C) | 760 | 140 | 14 |
| (D) | 690 | 120 | 16 |
| (E) | 900 | 150 | 12 |

51m. Based on the equation $\dot{V}_A = (V_T - V_D) \times RR$, the alveolar minute ventilation ($\dot{V}_A$) may be increased by all of the following *except*

(A) increasing the $V_T$

(B) decreasing the $V_T$

(C) decreasing the $V_D$

(D) increasing the $RR$

(E) increasing the $V_T$ and $RR$

CHAPTER

# 52
# Oxygen:Air (O₂:Air) Entrainment Ratio

## NOTES

This equation calculates the $O_2$:air entrainment ratio at any $F_IO_2$ between 21% and 99%.

In the equation shown, the 21 represents the oxygen fraction of room air. The 21 should not be rounded off to 20 in calculations involving $F_IO_2$ of less than 30% because rounding off can cause erroneous results.

To find the total flow of a venturi device, simply add the $O_2$:air ratio and then multiply the sum by the oxygen flow rate. For example, the $O_2$:air ratio for 28% oxygen is 1:10, and therefore the total flow of a 28% oxygen venturi device running at 4 L/min of oxygen is $(1 + 10) \times 4$ or 44 L/min.

## EQUATION

$$O_2:air = 1 : \frac{100 - F_IO_2}{F_IO_2 - 21}$$

$O_2$:air  :   Oxygen:air entrainment ratio

$F_IO_2$   :   Inspired oxygen concentration in %

## EXAMPLE 1

Find the $O_2$:air ratio of 28% oxygen.

$$O_2:air = 1 : \frac{100 - 28}{28 - 21}$$

$$= 1 : \frac{72}{7}$$

$$= 1 : 10.3 \text{ or } 1{:}10$$

At 28% oxygen, every 1 unit of oxygen is mixed with 10 units of air. See Fig. 35 for the progression of a "tick-tack-toe" method to solve this problem.

| 21  — 100<br>— $F_IO_2$ —<br>— — — | 21  — 100<br>— 28 —<br>— — — | 21  — 100<br>— 28 —<br>72  /  −7 = 10.3 |
|---|---|---|
| Set up tick-tack-toe as above. | To find $O_2$: air ratio for 28% oxygen, write 28% in the $F_IO_2$ block. | Subtract the numbers diagonally. Divide the resulting numbers (72/7). The ratio is 1:10.3 or 1:10. [Disregard the minus sign] |

**Figure 35**  *A "tick-tack-toe" method to solve for $O_2$ :air entrainment ratio of 28% oxygen. 21 represents the percentage of oxygen in room air, and 100 represents the percentage of oxygen from a pure oxygen source.*

**EXAMPLE 2**   Find the O$_2$:air ratio of 70% oxygen.

$$O_2 : air = 1 : \frac{100 - 70}{70 - 21}$$

$$= 1 : \frac{30}{49}$$

$$= 1 : 0.61 \text{ or } 1{:}0.6$$

At 70% oxygen, every 1 unit of oxygen is mixed with 0.6 units of air. See Fig. 36 for the progession of another "tick-tack-toe" method to solve this problem.

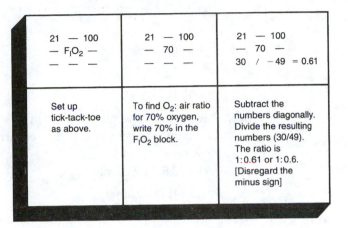

**Figure 36**   *A "tick-tack-toe" method to solve for O$_2$:air entrainment ratio of 28% oxygen. 21 represents the percentage of oxygen in room air, and 100 represents the percentage of oxygen from a pure oxygen source.*

**EXERCISE 1**   Find the O$_2$:air ratio of a 24% oxygen venturi device.

[Answer: O$_2$:air = 1 : 25.33 or 1:25]

**EXERCISE 2**   What is the total flow of this 24% oxygen venturi device if an oxygen flow rate of 4 L/min is used?

[Answer: Total flow rate = 104 L/min]

**REFERENCES**   Barnes; White

## Self-Assessment Questions

52a.  The oxygen:air entrainment ratio for 60% oxygen is
  (A) 1 : 0.7
  (B) 1 : 1
  (C) 1 : 3
  (D) 1 : 5
  (E) 1 : 7

52b.  Calculate the O$_2$:air ratio of 30% oxygen.
  (A) 1 : 7.8
  (B) 1 : 8.1
  (C) 1 : 8.9
  (D) 1 : 10
  (E) 1 : 12

52c.  An oxygen flow rate of 12 L/min is used on a 60% venturi mask. What is the O$_2$:air entrainment ratio of the venturi mask? What is the total flow at this oxygen flow rate?
  (A) 1 : 0.6; 19.2 L/min
  (B) 1 : 1; 24 L/min
  (C) 1 : 1; 26.4 L/min
  (D) 1 : 1.6; 31.2 L/min
  (E) 1 : 1.6; 36 L/min

52d.  What is the total flow of a 40% venturi mask running at 6 L/min of oxygen?
  (A) 12.6 L/min
  (B) 18.2 L/min
  (C) 24.9 L/min
  (D) 28.5 L/min
  (E) 32.7 L/min

52e.  If a patient is using a 40% venturi mask and a total flow of 36 L/min is desired, what should be the minimum oxygen flow rate?
  (A) 6 L/min
  (B) 7 L/min
  (C) 8 L/min
  (D) 9 L/min
  (E) 10 L/min

52f.  A venturi aerosol unit is used to deliver 50% oxygen with aerosol to a patient. What is the oxygen:air ratio at this $F_IO_2$? What is the total flow at 6 L/min of oxygen?
  (A) 1 : 1.5; 13.8 L/min
  (B) 1 : 1.5; 15 L/min
  (C) 1 : 1.7; 16.2 L/min
  (D) 1 : 1.7; 17.4 L/min
  (E) 1 : 2.1; 18.6 L/min

52g.  A patient is receiving 35% oxygen via a venturi mask at 6 L/min of oxygen. What is the total flow available to this patient? If the patient's minute ventilation is 11 L/min, would the total flow of this venturi setup satisfy the patient's ventilation needs?

(A)  12.8 L/min; no

(B)  27.6 L/min; yes

(C)  27.6 L/min; no

(D)  33.8 L/min; yes

(E)  33.8 L/min; no

# *53*
# Oxygen Consumption ($\dot{V}O_2$) and Index ($\dot{V}O_2$ Index)

As shown in the example, a person who has a cardiac output ($\dot{Q}_T$) of 5 L/min and an arterial–mixed venous oxygen content difference [$C(a-\overline{v})O_2$] of 4 vol% will consume 200 mL of oxygen per minute. Under normal conditions, oxygen consumption ($\dot{V}O_2$) is directly related to $\dot{Q}_T$ and [$C(a-\overline{v})O_2$].

Conditions leading to higher oxygen consumption (e.g., exercise) cause the cardiac output ($\dot{Q}_T$) to increase. If the cardiac output fails to keep up with the oxygen consumption needs, the $C(a-\overline{v})O_2$ increases. Some factors that increase oxygen consumption are listed in Table 5.

On the other hand, conditions leading to lower oxygen consumption (e.g., skeletal relaxation) cause the cardiac output to decrease. If the cardiac output provides an oxygen level higher than that required or consumed by the body, the $C(a-\overline{v})O_2$ decreases. Some factors that decrease oxygen consumption are listed in Table 6.

Oxygen consumption index ($\dot{V}O_2$ index) is used to normalize oxygen consumption measurements among patients of varying body size. The example shows that a $\dot{V}O_2$ index of 143 mL/min/m$^2$ is normal for an average-sized person ($BSA = 1.4$ m$^2$) but low ($\dot{V}O_2$ index = 100 mL/min/m$^2$) for a large person ($BSA = 2$ m$^2$).

## EQUATION 1

$$\dot{V}O_2 = \dot{Q}_T \times C(a-\overline{v})O_2$$

## EQUATION 2

$$\dot{V}O_2 \text{ index} = \frac{\dot{V}O_2}{BSA}$$

| | | |
|---|---|---|
| $\dot{V}O_2$ | : | Oxygen consumption in mL/min; oxygen uptake |
| $\dot{V}O_2$ index | : | Oxygen consumption index in L/min/m$^2$ |
| $\dot{Q}_T$ | : | Cardiac output in L/min; $CO$ |
| $C(a-\overline{v})O_2$ | : | Arterial–mixed venous oxygen content difference in vol% |
| $BSA$ | : | Body surface area in m$^2$ |

## NORMAL VALUES

$$\dot{V}O_2 = 200 \text{ to } 350 \text{ mL/min}$$
$$\dot{V}O_2 \text{ index} = 125 \text{ to } 165 \text{ mL/min/m}^2$$

## EXAMPLE

Given: 
$$\dot{Q}_T = 5 \text{ L/min}$$
$$C(a-\overline{v})O_2 = 4 \text{ vol\%}$$
$$BSA = 1.4 \text{ m}^2 \text{ (patient 1) and}$$
$$BSA = 2 \text{ m}^2 \text{ (patient 2)}$$

Calculate the oxygen consumption and oxygen consumption indices for both patients.

$$\dot{V}O_2 = \dot{Q}_T \times C(a-\overline{v})O_2$$
$$= 5 \text{ L/min} \times 4 \text{ vol\%}$$
$$= 5 \text{ L/min} \times 0.04$$
$$= 0.2 \text{ L/min}$$
$$= 200 \text{ mL/min}$$

$$\dot{V}O_2 \text{ index for patient 1} = \frac{\dot{V}O_2}{BSA \text{ of patient 1}}$$
$$= \frac{200}{1.4}$$
$$= 143 \text{ mL/min/m}^2$$

$$\dot{V}O_2 \text{ index for patient 2} = \frac{\dot{V}O_2}{BSA \text{ of patient 2}}$$

$$= \frac{200}{2}$$

$$= 100 \text{ mL/min/m}^2$$

---

**TABLE 5. Factors That Increase Oxygen Consumption**

Exercise

Seizures

Shivering in postoperative patient

Hyperthermia

---

From Des Jardins, T.R., *Cardiopulmonary Anatomy and Physiology: Essentials for Respiratory Care,* 3rd ed. Albany, NY: Delmar Publishers, 1998.

---

## EXERCISE

Given: $\dot{Q}_T = 4.5 \text{ L/min}$

$C(a - \bar{v})O_2 = 5 \text{ vol\%}$

$BSA = 1.2 \text{ m}^2$

Calculate the oxygen consumption and oxygen consumption indices. Are they within normal limits?

[Answer: $\dot{V}O_2 = 225 \text{ mL/min}$; normal. $\dot{V}O_2$ index = 187.5 mL/min/m$^2$; abnormal]

---

**TABLE 6. Factors That Decrease Oxygen Consumption**

Skeletal relaxation (e.g., induced by drugs)

Peripheral shunting (e.g., sepsis, trauma)

Certain poisons (e.g., cyanide prevents cellular metabolism)

Hypothermia

---

From Des Jardins, T.R., *Cardiopulmonary Anatomy and Physiology: Essentials for Respiratory Care,* 3rd ed. Albany: NY: Delmar Publishers, 1998.

---

## REFERENCES

Des Jardins; Kacmarek

## SEE

*Arterial–Mixed Venous Oxygen Content Difference [C(a − v̄)O₂]; Cardiac Output (CO): Fick's Estimated Method; Appendix F, DuBois Body Surface Chart.*

## Self-Assessment Questions

53a. Oxygen consumption ($\dot{V}O_2$) in mL/min is calculated by

(A) $\dot{Q}_T \times C(a-v)O_2$

(B) $\dfrac{\dot{Q}_T}{C(a-v)O_2}$

(C) $\dot{Q}_T + C(a-v)O_2$

(D) $\dot{Q}_T - C(a-v)O_2$

(E) $\dfrac{C(a-v)O_2}{\dot{Q}_T}$

53b. The normal oxygen consumption ($\dot{V}O_2$) rate for an adult is between

(A) 80 and 120 mL/min

(B) 120 and 200 mL/min

(C) 200 and 350 mL/min

(D) 350 and 500 mL/min

(E) 500 and 850 mL/min

53c. Given: cardiac output $\dot{Q}_T$ = 5.0 L/min, arterial–mixed venous oxygen content difference [$C(a-\bar{v})O_2$] = 3.5 vol%, body surface area (*BSA*) = 1.6 m$^2$. Calculate the oxygen consumption ($\dot{V}O_2$) rate.

(A) 130 mL/min

(B) 145 mL/min

(C) 160 mL/min

(D) 175 mL/min

(E) 200 mL/min

53d. A patient whose body surface area is 1.4 m$^2$ has a measured oxygen consumption ($\dot{V}O_2$) of 200 mL/min. What is the calculated oxygen consumption index ($\dot{V}O_2$ index)?

(A) 117 mL/min/m$^2$

(B) 120 mL/min/m$^2$

(C) 125 mL/min/m$^2$

(D) 130 mL/min/m$^2$

(E) 143 mL/min/m$^2$

53e. Given: cardiac output $\dot{Q}_T$ = 3.6 L/min, arterial–mixed venous oxygen content difference [$C(a-\bar{v})O_2$] = 4.0 vol%, body surface area (*BSA*) = 1.0 m$^2$. Calculate the oxygen consumption ($\dot{V}O_2$) and its index ($\dot{V}O_2$ index).

(A) 132 mL/min; 144 mL/min/m$^2$

(B) 144 mL/min; 144 mL/min/m$^2$

(C) 150 mL/min; 150 mL/min/m$^2$

(D) 165 mL/min; 150 mL/min/m$^2$

(E) 177 mL/min; 165 mL/min/m$^2$

53f. Which of the following measurements has the highest oxygen consumption rate?

| | $\dot{Q}_T$ (L/min) | $C(a-\bar{v})O_2$ (vol%) |
|---|---|---|
| (A) | 3.4 | 5.3 |
| (B) | 3.9 | 4.9 |
| (C) | 4.2 | 5.0 |
| (D) | 4.7 | 4.1 |
| (E) | 5.5 | 3.9 |

53g. Which of the following measurements has the highest oxygen consumption index?

| | $Q_T$ (L/min) | $C(a-\overline{v})O_2$ (vol%) | Body surface area ($m^2$) |
|---|---|---|---|
| (A) | 3.4 | 5.3 | 1.6 |
| (B) | 3.9 | 4.9 | 1.5 |
| (C) | 4.2 | 5.0 | 1.7 |
| (D) | 4.7 | 4.1 | 1.9 |
| (E) | 5.5 | 3.9 | 2.1 |

# CHAPTER

# 54

# Oxygen Content: Arterial ($C_aO_2$)

## NOTES

$C_aO_2$ reflects the overall oxygen carrying capacity of arterial blood. The major determinants of oxygen content are the hemoglobin (Hb) level and the oxygen saturation ($S_aO_2$). In normal arterial blood gases, the amount of dissolved $O_2$ contributes only about 0.3 vol% to the oxygen content of 20 vol% (Fig. 37).

A low Hb level (e.g., anemia) or a low $O_2$ saturation (e.g., hypoxia) will significantly lower the arterial oxygen content. On the other hand, a high Hb level (e.g., polycythemia) or high $O_2$ saturation (e.g., hyperoxia) will raise the arterial oxygen content.

## EQUATION

$$C_aO_2 = (Hb \times 1.34 \times S_aO_2) + (P_aO_2 \times 0.003)$$

| | | |
|---|---|---|
| $C_aO_2$ | : | Arterial oxygen content in vol% |
| Hb | : | Hemoglobin content in g% |
| $S_aO_2$ | : | Arterial oxygen saturation in % |
| $P_aO_2$ | : | Arterial oxygen tension in mm Hg |

## NORMAL VALUE

16 to 20 vol%

## EXAMPLE

Given: Hb  = 15 g%

$S_aO_2$ = 98%

$P_aO_2$ = 100 mg Hg

Calculate the arterial oxygen content.

$$\begin{aligned} C_aO_2 &= (Hb \times 1.34 \times S_aO_2) + (P_aO_2 \times 0.003) \\ &= (15 \times 1.34 \times 98\%) + (100 \times 0.003) \\ &= 19.70 + 0.3 \\ &= 20 \text{ vol\%} \end{aligned}$$

## EXERCISE

Given: Hb  = 10 g%

$S_aO_2$ = 80%

$P_aO_2$ = 60 mm Hg

Calculate the $C_aO_2$.

[Answer: $C_aO_2 = 10.9$ vol%]

## REFERENCES

Shapiro (1); Malley

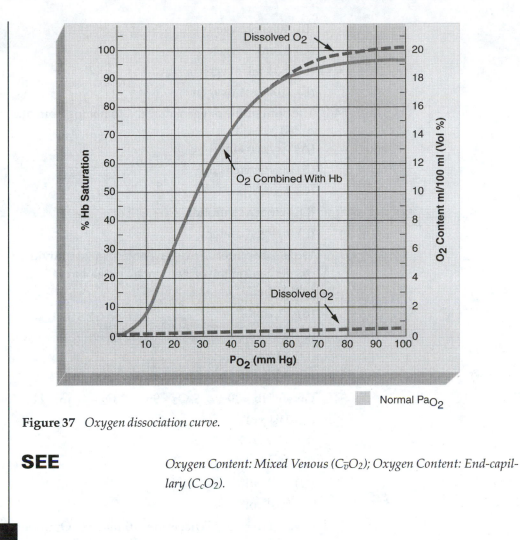

**Figure 37**  *Oxygen dissociation curve.*

**SEE**  *Oxygen Content: Mixed Venous ($C_{\bar{v}}O_2$); Oxygen Content: End-capillary ($C_cO_2$).*

# Self-Assessment Questions

54a. When the $P_aO_2$ is 50 mm Hg, the amount of oxygen dissolved in 100 mL of blood is about
   (A) 0.05 mL
   (B) 0.10 mL
   (C) 0.15 mL
   (D) 0.20 mL
   (E) 0.25 mL

54b. The amount of oxygen bound to the hemoglobin (Hb) is normally calculated by using the equation
   (A) $Hb \times 1.34 + P_aO_2 \times 0.003$
   (B) $Hb \times 1.34$
   (C) $Hb \times 1.34 \times S_aO_2$
   (D) $Hb \times S_aO_2$
   (E) $Hb \times P_aO_2 \times S_aO_2$

54c. In 100 mL of blood, I g of hemoglobin when fully saturated with oxygen can carry
   (A) 100 mL oxygen

(B) 40 mL oxygen

(C) 47 mL oxygen

(D) 1.34 mL oxygen

(E) 0.003 mL oxygen

54d. The sum of the oxygen attached to hemoglobin and that dissolved in plasma is called

(A) oxygen affinity

(B) oxygen tension

(C) $P_{50}$

(D) oxygen saturation

(E) oxygen content

54e. What is the arterial oxygen content of an individual who has a $P_aO_2$ of 300 torr, oxygen saturation of 99%, and hemoglobin of 16 g?

(A) 22.1 mL

(B) 21.7 mL

(C) 21.4 mL

(D) 19.6 mL

(E) 0.9 mL

54f. Given: Hb = 10 g%, $S_aO_2$ = 95%, $P_aO_2$ = 60 mm Hg. The calculated $C_aO_2$ is

(A) 11.1 vol%

(B) 12.9 vol%

(C) 15.6 vol%

(D) 17.3 vol%

(E) 19.0 vol%

54g. Given: Hb = 15 g. What is the estimated $C_aO_2$ under normal conditions?

(A) 7 vol%

(B) 10 vol%

(C) 15 vol%

(D) 18 vol%

(E) 20 vol%

54h. What is the arterial oxygen content ($C_aO_2$) of a patient who has a $P_aO_2$ of 100 mm Hg, oxygen saturation of 98%, and a hemoglobin of 12 g/100 mL of blood?

(A) 14 vol%

(B) 15 vol%

(C) 16 vol%

(D) 17 vol%

(E) 18 vol%

54i. Given: Hb = 10 g%, $S_aO_2$ = 90%, $P_aO_2$ = 80 mm Hg. Calculate the arterial oxygen content ($C_aO_2$).

(A) 10.2 vol%

(B) 11.1 vol%

(C) 12.3 vol%

(D) 13.4 vol%

(E) 20.1 vol%

54j.  A polycythemic patient has the following blood gas values: Hb = 17 g%, $S_aO_2$ = 90%, $P_aO_2$ = 60 mm Hg. Based on these results, what is the calculated arterial oxygen content ($C_aO_2$)?

(A)  19.4 vol%

(B)  19.6 vol%

(C)  20.5 vol%

(D)  20.7 vol%

(E)  22.8 vol%

54k.  Which of the following blood gas measurements has the lowest calculated arterial oxygen content ($C_aO_2$)?

|     | Hb (g%) | $S_aO_2$ (%) | $P_aO_2$ (mm Hg) |
|-----|---------|--------------|------------------|
| (A) | 13      | 98           | 100              |
| (B) | 15      | 70           | 55               |
| (C) | 16      | 80           | 76               |
| (D) | 14      | 85           | 82               |
| (E) | 15      | 82           | 78               |

54l.  The blood gas measurements of a patient recovering from massive blood loss are as follows: Hb = 8 g%, $S_aO_2$ = 98%, $P_aO_2$ = 100 mm Hg. What is the calculated $C_aO_2$? Is it normal?

(A)  10.1 vol%; normal

(B)  10.1 vol%; abnormal

(C)  10.5 vol%; normal

(D)  10.8 vol%; normal

(E)  10.8 vol%; abnormal

# CHAPTER

# *55*
# Oxygen Content: End-Capillary ($C_cO_2$)

## NOTES

$C_cO_2$ is a calculated value representing the best oxygen content possible at the pulmonary end-capillary level. It is used in other calculations such as shunt equation.

End-capillary oxygen content reflects the optimal oxygen carrying capacity of the cardiopulmonary system. The oxygen saturation is assumed to be 100%. The major determinant of $C_cO_2$ is the hemoglobin (Hb) level. A low Hb level (e.g., anemia) will significantly lower the end-capillary oxygen content.

## EQUATION

$$C_cO_2 = (Hb \times 1.34 \times S_aO_2) + (P_AO_2 \times 0.003)^*$$

$C_cO_2$ : End-capillary oxygen content in vol%
Hb : Hemoglobin content in g%
$S_aO_2$ : Arterial oxygen saturation, assumed to be 100% in $C_cO_2$ calculations
$P_AO_2$ : Alveolar oxygen tension in mm Hg, used in place of end-capillary $PO_2$ ($P_cO_2$)

## NORMAL VALUE

Varies according to the hemoglobin level and the $F_IO_2$.

## EXAMPLE

Given: Hb   = 15 g%
     $F_IO_2$   = 21% [$P_AO_2$ = 100 mm Hg]
Calculate the end-capillary oxygen content ($C_cO_2$).

$$
\begin{aligned}
C_cO_2 &= (Hb \times 1.34 \times S_aO_2) + (P_AO_2 \times 0.003) \\
&= (15 \times 1.34 \times 100\%) + (100 \times 0.003) \\
&= 20.1 + 0.3 \\
&= 20.4 \text{ vol\%}
\end{aligned}
$$

## EXERCISE

Given: Hb   = 10 g%
     $F_IO_2$   = 40% [From Appendix B: $P_AO_2$ = 235 mm Hg]
Calculate the $C_cO_2$.

[Answer: $C_cO_2$ = 14.11 vol%]

## REFERENCES

Shapiro (1); Malley

**SEE**    *Oxygen Content: Arterial ($C_aO_2$); Oxygen Content: Mixed Venous ($C_{\bar{v}}O_2$).*

*\*See: Appendix B: $P_AO_2$ at selected $F_IO_2$.*

## Self-Assessment Questions

55a. Which of the following calculations requires a $P_AO_2$ value?

(A) $C_{\bar{v}}O_2$

(B) $C_aO_2$

(C) $C_cO_2$

(D) $\dfrac{V_D}{V_T}$

(E) Oxygen:air entrainment ratio

55b. Given: Hb = 14 g%, $F_IO_2$ = 21% ($P_AO_2$ = 100 mm Hg). Calculate the end-capillary oxygen content ($C_cO_2$).

(A) 18.8 vol%

(B) 19.1 vol%

(C) 20.1 vol%

(D) 21 vol%

(E) insufficient information to calculate answer

55c. Given: Hb = 15 g%; $F_IO_2$ = 100% ($P_AO_2$ = 673 mm Hg). Calculate the end-capillary oxygen content ($C_cO_2$).

(A) 20.1 vol%

(B) 21.4 vol%

(C) 22.1 vol%

(D) 23.2 vol%

(E) $S_aO_2$ required to calculate answer

55d. Which of the following measurements has the highest calculated end-capillary oxygen content ($C_cO_2$)?

|     | Hb (g%) | $F_IO_2$ (%) | $P_AO_2$ (mm Hg) |
| --- | --- | --- | --- |
| (A) | 11 | 100 | 673 |
| (B) | 12 | 80 | 530 |
| (C) | 13 | 60 | 388 |
| (D) | 14 | 40 | 235 |
| (E) | 15 | 21 | 100 |

55e. A polycythemic patient who is recovering from coronary artery bypass surgery has the following measurements: Hb = 17 g%, $F_IO_2$ = 30% ($P_AO_2$ = 164 mm Hg). What is the calculated $C_cO_2$ for this patient?

(A) 20.1 vol%

(B) 21.9 vol%

(C) 22.8 vol%

(D) 23.3 vol%

(E) 26.5 vol%

# CHAPTER

# 56
# Oxygen Content: Mixed Venous ($C_{\bar{v}}O_2$)

## NOTE

Mixed venous oxygen content ($C_{\bar{v}}O_2$) reflects the overall oxygen level of the blood returning to the right heart. $C_{\bar{v}}O_2$ is affected by a number of factors. Low Hb level (e.g., anemia), low $O_2$ saturation (e.g., hypoxemia), decrease in cardiac output (e.g., congestive heart failure), or increase in metabolic rate (e.g., exercise) will significantly lower the $C_{\bar{v}}O_2$. Refer to Table 7 for factors that decrease the mixed venous oxygen content.

## EQUATION

$$C_{\bar{v}}O_2 = (\text{Hb} \times 1.34 \times S_{\bar{v}}O_2) + (P_{\bar{v}}O_2 \times 0.003)$$

$C_{\bar{v}}O_2$ : Mixed venous oxygen content in vol%

Hb : Hemoglobin content in g%

$S_{\bar{v}}O_2$ : Mixed venous oxygen saturation in vol%

$P_{\bar{v}}O_2$ : Mixed venous oxygen tension in mm Hg

## NORMAL VALUE

12 to 15 vol%

## EXAMPLE

Given: Hb $= 15\,\text{g}\%$

$\qquad S_{\bar{v}}O_2 = 70\%$

$\qquad P_{\bar{v}}O_2 = 35\,\text{mm Hg}$

Calculate the mixed venous oxygen content ($C_{\bar{v}}O_2$).

$\begin{aligned}
C_{\bar{v}}O_2 &= (\text{Hb} \times 1.34 \times S_{\bar{v}}O_2) + (P_{\bar{v}}O_2 \times 0.003) \\
&= (15 \times 1.34 \times 70\%) + (35 \times 0.003) \\
&= 14.07 + 0.11 \\
&= 14.18\,\text{vol}\%
\end{aligned}$

## EXERCISE

Given: Hb $= 12\,\text{g}\%$

$\qquad S_{\bar{v}}O_2 = 75\%$

$\qquad P_{\bar{v}}O_2 = 40\,\text{mm Hg}$

Calculate the $C_{\bar{v}}O_2$.

[Answer: $C_{\bar{v}}O_2 = 12.18$ vol%]

## REFERENCES

Shapiro (1); Malley

| **SEE** | *Oxygen Content: Arterial ($C_aO_2$); Oxygen Content: End-Capillary ($C_cO_2$).* |
|---|---|

---

**TABLE 7. Factors That Decrease $C_{\bar{v}}O_2$**

Low hemoglobin
Low $O_2$ saturation
Decreased cardiac output
Increased metabolic rate

---

# Self-Assessment Questions

56a. Given: Hb = 13 g%, $S_{\bar{v}}O_2$ = 70%, $P_{\bar{v}}O_2$ = 40 mm Hg. Calculate the mixed venous oxygen content ($C_{\bar{v}}O_2$).

(A) 12.3 vol%

(B) 12.9 vol%

(C) 13.6 vol%

(D) 14.2 vol%

(E) 14.8 vol%

56b. A sample obtained from the pulmonary artery has the following results: Hb = 14 g%, $S_{\bar{v}}O_2$ = 75%, $P_{\bar{v}}O_2$ = 40 mm Hg. Calculate the $C_{\bar{v}}O_2$. Is it normal?

(A) 12.3 vol%; abnormal

(B) 13.6 vol%; normal

(C) 13.6 vol%; abnormal

(D) 14.2 vol%; normal

(E) 14.2 vol%; abnormal

56c. Which of the following blood gas measurements has the lowest mixed venous oxygen content ($C_{\bar{v}}O_2$)?

|     | **Hb (g%)** | **$S_{\bar{v}}O_2$ (%)** | **$P_{\bar{v}}O_2$ (mm Hg)** |
|-----|-------------|--------------------------|------------------------------|
| (A) | 13          | 74                       | 30                           |
| (B) | 15          | 66                       | 34                           |
| (C) | 14          | 75                       | 38                           |
| (D) | 14          | 72                       | 36                           |
| (E) | 15          | 69                       | 35                           |

56d. An anemic patient who is admitted for shortness of breath has the following measurements: Hb = 9 g%, $S_{\bar{v}}O_2$ = 73%; $P_{\bar{v}}O_2$ = 38 mm Hg. What is the calculated $C_{\bar{v}}O_2$ for this patient? Is it normal?

(A) 8.9 vol%; abnormal

(B) 8.9 vol%; normal

(C) 12.1 vol%; abnormal

(D) 12.1 vol%; normal

(E) 20.1 vol%; normal

# CHAPTER

# *57*

# Oxygen Duration of E Cylinder

## NOTES

In this type of oxygen duration calculation, it is essential to remember the conversion factor (0.28) for the E oxygen cylinder (Appendix K). This conversion factor (0.28 L/psig) is derived by dividing the volume of oxygen (622 L) by the gauge pressure (2200 psig) of a full E cylinder (622 L/2200 psig = 0.283 L/psig).

The 622 L comes from 22 ft$^3$ × 28.3 L/ft$^3$ since an E cylinder holds about 22 ft$^3$ of compressed oxygen and each ft$^3$ of compressed oxygen gives 28.3 L of gaseous oxygen.

To change minutes to hours and minutes, simply divide the minutes by 60. The whole number represents the hours, and the remainder is the minutes.

When a calculator is used, the number in front of the decimal is the hours. The number after the decimal, including the decimal point, should be multiplied by 60 to obtain minutes.

## EQUATION

$$\text{Duration of E} = \frac{0.28 \times \text{psig}}{\text{Liter flow}}$$

Duration of E  :  Duration of oxygen remaining in an E cylinder in minutes

psig  :  Gauge pressure, pounds per square inch

Liter flow  :  Oxygen flow rate in L/min

## EXAMPLE

Given: E oxygen cylinder with 2000 psig

Oxygen flow = 5 L/min

A. Calculate how long the cylinder will last until 0 psig.

$$\begin{aligned}
\text{Duration} &= \frac{0.28 \times \text{psig}}{\text{Liter flow}} \\
&= \frac{0.28 \times 2000}{5} \\
&= \frac{560}{5} \\
&= 112 \text{ min or } 1 \text{ hr } 52 \text{ min}
\end{aligned}$$

B. Calculate how long the cylinder will last until the pressure reaches 500 psig.

$$\begin{aligned}
\text{Duration to 500 psig} &= \frac{0.28 \times (\text{psig} - 500)}{\text{Liter flow}} \\
&= \frac{0.28 \times (2000 - 500)}{5} \\
&= \frac{0.28 \times 1500}{5} \\
&= \frac{420}{5} \\
&= 84 \text{ min or } 1 \text{ hr } 24 \text{ min}
\end{aligned}$$

**EXERCISE 1**    Given: E oxygen cylinder with 2200 psig
                        Oxygen flow rate = 5 L/min
How long will the oxygen remain in this cylinder at this flow rate until the cylinder reaches 0 psig?

[Answer: Duration = 123 min or 2 hr 3 min]

**EXERCISE 2**

Given: E oxygen cylinder with 1600 psig
Oxygen flow rate = 2 L/min
Calculate the duration of oxygen remaining in this cylinder (to 0 psig). How long will it last until 500 psig?

[Answer: Duration = 224 min or 3 hr 44 min;
Duration to 500 psig = 154 min or 2 hr 34 min.]

**REFERENCES**    Scanlan; White

## Self-Assessment Questions

57a. Given: E oxygen cylinder with 2000 psig, oxygen flow = 2 L/min. Calculate the duration until the pressure reaches 0 psig at this flow rate.
   (A) 3 hr 55 min
   (B) 4 hr 15 min
   (C) 4 hr 30 min
   (D) 4 hr 40 min
   (E) 4 hr 55 min

57b. An E oxygen cylinder is full at 2200 psig. If a flow rate is set at 2 L/min, how long will this cylinder last until it reaches a gauge pressure of 200 psig?
   (A) 1 hr 20 min
   (B) 3 hr 30 min
   (C) 4 hr 40 min
   (D) 5 hr 10 min
   (E) 52 hr 10 min

57c.  An E oxygen cylinder with 1400 psig is available for patient transport. At an oxygen flow rate of 2 L/min, what is the maximum travel time the patient can rely on until this cylinder reaches 500 psig?

(A) 1 hr

(B) 1 hr 10 min

(C) 2 hr 6 min

(D) 3 hr 16 min

(E) 4 hr 12 min

57d.  An E oxygen cylinder with 1800 psig is being used at a flow rate of 3 L/min. How long will the cylinder last until the pressure reaches 0 psig? Until the pressure reaches 200 psig?

(A) 2 hr 48 min; 2 hr 29 min

(B) 2 hr 48 min; 2 hr 10 min

(C) 3 hr 20 min; 3 hr 1 min

(D) 3 hr 20 min; 2 hr 42 min

(E) 3 hr 55 min; 3 hr 36 min

57e.  At its respective flow rate, which of the following E cylinders would provide the longest duration of oxygen?

| | psig | Flow (L/min) |
| --- | --- | --- |
| (A) | 500 | 1 |
| (B) | 700 | 1.5 |
| (C) | 800 | 2 |
| (D) | 900 | 2.5 |
| (E) | 1400 | 3 |

# CHAPTER

# *58*

# Oxygen Duration of H or K Cylinder

## *NOTES*

In this type of oxygen duration calculation, it is essential to remember the conversion factor (3.14) for the H or K oxygen cylinder (Appendix K). This conversion factor (3.14 L/psig) is derived by dividing the volume of oxygen (6900 L) by the gauge pressure (2200 psig) of a full H or K cylinder:

$$\frac{6900 \text{ L}}{2200 \text{ psig}} = 3.136 \text{ L/psig.}$$

The 6900 L comes from 224 $\text{ft}^3 \times 28.3$ L/$\text{ft}^3$ since H and K cylinders hold about 244 $\text{ft}^3$ of compressed oxygen, and each $\text{ft}^3$ of compressed oxygen gives 28.3 L of gaseous oxygen.

To change minutes to hours and minutes, simply divide the minutes by 60. The whole number represents the hours, and the remainder is the minutes.

When a calculator is used to divide, the number in front of the decimal is the hours. The number after the decimal, including the decimal point, should be multiplied by 60 to obtain minutes.

## EQUATION

$$\text{Duration of K} = \frac{3.14 \times \text{psig}}{\text{Liter flow}}$$

Duration of K  :  Duration of oxygen remaining in an H or K cylinder in minutes

psig  :  Gauge pressure, pounds per square inch

Liter flow  :  Oxygen flow rate in L/min

## EXAMPLE

Given: K oxygen cylinder with 1000 psig

Oxygen flow = 5 L/min

A. Calculate how long the cylinder will last until 0 psig.

$$\begin{aligned}
\text{Duration} &= \frac{3.14 \times \text{psig}}{\text{Liter flow}} \\
&= \frac{3.14 \times 1000}{5} \\
&= \frac{3140}{5} \\
&= 628 \text{ min or 10 hr 28 min}
\end{aligned}$$

B. Calculate how long the cylinder will last until the pressure reaches 200 psig.

$$\begin{aligned}
\text{Duration to 200 psig} &= \frac{3.14 \times (\text{psig} - 200)}{\text{Liter flow}} \\
&= \frac{3.14 \times (1000 - 200)}{5} \\
&= \frac{3.14 \times 800}{5} \\
&= \frac{2512}{5} \\
&= 502 \text{ min or 8 hr 22 min}
\end{aligned}$$

**EXERCISE**

Given: K oxygen cylinder with 2200 psig
Oxygen flow rate = 2 L/min
Calculate the duration of oxygen remaining in this cylinder.
How long will the cylinder last until it reaches 200 psig?

[Answer: Duration = 3454 min or 57 hr 34 min;
Duration to 200 psig = 3140 min or 52 hr 20 min]

**REFERENCES** Scanlan; White

## Self-Assessment Questions

58a. A K oxygen cylinder has a guage pressure of 1600 psig and is running at a flow rate of 5 L/min. After about how many hours will the pressure reach 0 psig at this flow rate?
   (A) 8
   (B) 10
   (C) 12
   (D) 14
   (E) 16

58b. Given: K oxygen cylinder with 2200 psig, oxygen flow = 5 L/min. Calculate the duration until the pressure reaches 0 psig at this flow rate.
   (A) 2 hr
   (B) 22 hr
   (C) 23 hr
   (D) 24 hr
   (E) 205 hr

58c. Given: K oxygen cylinder with 1200 psig, oxygen flow rate = 2 L/min. Calculate the duration of oxygen remaining in this cylinder until it reaches 200 psig.
   (A) 16 hr 15 min
   (B) 18 hr
   (C) 20 hr 30 min
   (D) 26 hr 10 min
   (E) 52 hr 20 min

58d. A K oxygen cylinder has a gauge reading of 1700 psig. How long will this cylinder last until it reaches 500 psig at an oxygen flow rate of 2 L/min?
   (A) 30 hr 16 min
   (B) 31 hr 24 min
   (C) 32 hr 10 min
   (D) 33 hr 42 min
   (E) 44 hr 29 min

58e. A K oxygen cylinder with 2000 psig is being used at a flow rate of 3 L/min. How long will the cylinder last until the pressure reaches 0 psig? Until the pressure reaches 500 psig?

(A) 29 hr 35 min; 18 hr 8 min

(B) 29 hr 35 min; 21 hr 12 min

(C) 34 hr 53 min; 24 hr 26 min

(D) 34 hr 53 min; 26 hr 10 min

(E) 36 hr 22 min; 28 hr 34 min

58f. During the last oxygen rounds at 10 P.M., a K oxygen cylinder has a gauge reading of 800 psig and the oxygen flow was set at 5 L/min. At this oxygen flow rate, about what time next morning will the gauge reading reach 500 psig?

(A) 1 A.M.

(B) 2 A.M.

(C) 3 A.M.

(D) 6 A.M.

(E) 8 A.M.

58g. Which of the following K cylinders would provide the longest duration of oxygen at its respective oxygen flow rate?

|  | psig | Flow (L/min) |
|---|---|---|
| (A) | 600 | 2 |
| (B) | 700 | 2.5 |
| (C) | 800 | 3 |
| (D) | 900 | 3.5 |
| (E) | 1000 | 4 |

# CHAPTER

# *59*

# Oxygen Duration of Liquid System

*NOTES*

In this type of oxygen duration calculation, it is essential to remember the conversion factor (344 L/lb) for the liquid oxygen cylinders. This conversion factor comes from 860/2.5 = 344 (Fig. 38). Liquid oxygen expands about 860 times to become gaseous oxygen, and it weighs 2.5 lb/L.

If the net weight of liquid oxygen is not shown, one can compute it by weighing the cylinder and liquid oxygen and subtracting the weight of the empty cylinder.

To change minutes to hours and minutes, simply divide minutes by 60. The whole number represents the hours, and the remainder is the minutes.

When a calculator is used to divide, the number in front of the decimal is the hours. The number after the decimal, including the decimal point, should be multiplied by 60 to get minutes.

The calculated duration does not account for the amount of liquid oxygen lost by normal evaporation. The evaporative rate of liquid oxygen ranges from 1 to 1.8 lb (0.4 to 0.72 liquid liters or 344 to 619 gaseous liters) per day.

## EQUATION 1

> When the liquid weight is known:

$$\text{Duration} = \frac{344 \times \text{Liquid weight}}{\text{Flow}}$$

| | | |
|---|---|---|
| Duration | : | Duration of oxygen remaining in a *liquid* $O_2$ cylinder, in min |
| 344 | : | A conversion factor, in L/lb |
| Liquid weight | : | The *net weight* of liquid oxygen in lb |
| Flow | : | Oxygen flow rate in L/min |

## EXAMPLE 1

If the net weight of liquid oxygen in a cylinder is 2 lb and the patient is using the contents at 1 L/min, how long will the liquid oxygen last?

$$\text{Duration} = \frac{344 \times \text{Liquid weight}}{\text{Flow}}$$

$$= \frac{344 \times 2}{1}$$

$$= \frac{688}{1}$$

$$= 688 \text{ min or } 11 \text{ hr } 28 \text{ min}$$

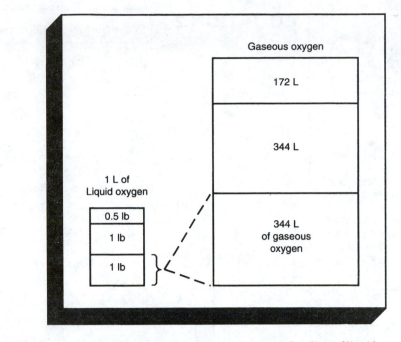

**Figure 38** *Volume relationship of liquid and gaseous oxygen. One liter of liquid oxygen weighs about 2.5 lbs. One pound of liquid oxygen equals 344 L of gaseous oxygen.*

**EXERCISE**    If the net weight of liquid oxygen in a cylinder is 2.5 lb, how long will the liquid oxygen last if the oxygen flow is running at 2 L/min?

[Answer: Duration = 430 min or 7 hr 10 min]

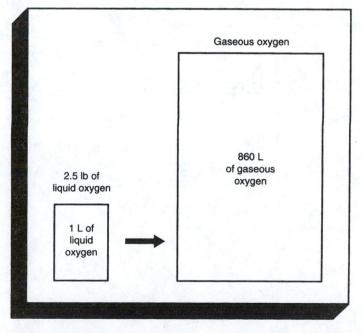

**Figure 39** *Volume relationship of liquid and gaseous oxygen. One liter of liquid oxygen weighs about 2.5 lbs and is equal to 860 L of gaseous oxygen.*

*NOTES*

One liter of liquid oxygen expands to about 860 L of gaseous oxygen (Fig. 39). Therefore, the liquid capacity is converted to gaseous capacity by multiplying the liquid capacity by 860.

To change minutes to hours and minutes, simply divide minutes by 60. The whole number represents the hours, and the remainder is the minutes.

When a calculator is used to divide, the number in front of the decimal is the hours. The number after the decimal, including the decimal point, should be multiplied by 60 to get minutes.

The calculated duration does not account for the amount of liquid oxygen lost by normal evaporation. The evaporative rate of liquid oxygen ranges from 1 to 1.8 lb (0.4 to 0.72 liquid liters of 344 to 619 gaseous liters) per day.

## EQUATION 2

When the gauge fraction is known:

$$\text{Duration} = \frac{\text{Capacity} \times 860 \times \text{Gauge fraction}}{\text{Flow}}$$

| Duration | : | Duration of oxygen remaining in a *liquid* $O_2$ cylinder, in min |
| Capacity | : | Capacity of liquid oxygen in cylinder, in L |
| 860 | : | Factor to convert liquid to gaseous oxygen, in L |
| Gauge fraction | : | Fractional reading of cylinder content |
| Flow | : | Oxygen flow rate in L/min |

## EXAMPLE 2

A portable liquid oxygen cylinder has a liquid capacity of 0.60 L. What is the gaseous capacity?

$$\begin{aligned}
\text{Gaseous capacity} &= \text{Liquid capacity} \times 860 \\
&= 0.60 \times 860 \\
&= 516 \text{ L}
\end{aligned}$$

## EXAMPLE 3

If the capacity of a liquid oxygen cylinder is 2.0 L and the gauge reading of the cylinder indicates it is $\frac{1}{3}$ full, how long will the liquid oxygen last if the flow is at 2 L/min?

$$\begin{aligned}
\text{Duration} &= \frac{\text{Capacity} \times 860 \times \text{Gauge fraction}}{\text{Flow}} \\
&= \frac{2 \times 860 \times \frac{1}{3}}{2} \\
&= \frac{1720 \times \frac{1}{3}}{2} \\
&= \frac{573}{2} \\
&= 287 \text{ min or 4 hr 47 min}
\end{aligned}$$

## EXERCISE

If the capacity of a liquid oxygen cylinder is 1.8 L and the gauge reading indicates it is $\frac{1}{2}$ full, how long will the liquid oxygen last if the oxygen flow is at 1 L/min?

[Answer: Duration = 774 min or 12 hr 54 min]

## REFERENCE

McPherson

## Self-Assessment Questions

59a. One pound of liquid oxygen can be expanded to become how many liters of gaseous oxygen?
(A) 2.5 L

(B) 344 L

(C) 500 L

(D) 860 L

(E) 960 L

59b. One liter of liquid oxygen weighs _____ pounds, and each liter can be expanded to become _____ liters of gaseous oxygen.
(A) 2 lb; 100 L

(B) 2 lb; 344 L

(C) 2.5 lb; 500 L

(D) 2.5 lb; 860 L

(E) 3 lb; 860 L

59c. Given: net weight of liquid oxygen in a cylinder = 4 lb. How long will the liquid oxygen last if the oxygen flow rate is 2 L/min?
(A) 6 hr 33 min

(B) 8 hr

(C) 10 hr

(D) 11 hr 28 min

(E) 26 hr 20 min

59d. The net weight of liquid oxygen in a cylinder is 3 lb. If a patient is using 2 L/min of oxygen on a continuous basis, how long will the liquid oxygen last?
(A) 7 hr 43 min

(B) 7 hr 50 min

(C) 8 hr 6 min

(D) 8 hr 36 min

(E) 8 hr 55 min

59e. A portable liquid oxygen cylinder has a net weight of 1.5 lb. At a flow rate of 1.5 L/min of oxygen, how long will it last until the portable system needs refilling?
(A) 4 hr 23 min

(B) 4 hr 45 min

(C) 5 hr 13 min

(D) 5 hr 30 min

(E) 5 hr 44 min

59f. The net weight remaining in a stationary liquid oxygen system is 10 lb, and the home care patient is using it 8 hr per day during sleep at a flow rate of 1 L/min. Based on this usage, about how many days will this liquid oxygen system last?
(A) 6 days

(B) 7 days

(C) 8 days

(D) 9 days

(E) 10 days

59g. If the capacity of a full liquid oxygen cylinder is 0.42 L, how long will the liquid oxygen last at a flow rate of 1 L/min?
(A) 6 hr 1 min
(B) 7 hr 16 min
(C) 8 hr
(D) 9 hr 25 min
(E) 16 hr 10 min

59h. A portable liquid oxygen cylinder has a liquid capacity of 0.49 L. What is the gaseous capacity?
(A) 387 L
(B) 403 L
(C) 421 L
(D) 452 L
(E) 504 L

59i. The capacity of a portable liquid oxygen cylinder is 2 L, and the gauge reading indicates it is $\frac{1}{2}$ full. If a patient is using 2 L/min of oxygen on a continuous basis, how long will the liquid oxygen last?
(A) 7 hr 10 min
(B) 7 hr 45 min
(C) 8 hr 36 min
(D) 9 hr 24 min
(E) 9 hr 55 min

59j. The capacity of a stationary home liquid oxygen system is 25.5 L, and it is $\frac{1}{4}$ full. If a patient is using 1.5 L/min of oxygen on a continuous basis, about how many hours will this liquid system last?
(A) 40 hr
(B) 50 hr
(C) 60 hr
(D) 70 hr
(E) 80 hr

59k. The liquid capacity of a full stationary liquid oxygen system is 37 L, and the home care patient is using it 8 hr per day during sleep at a flow rate of 2 L/min. Based on this usage, about how many days will this liquid oxygen system last?
(A) 5 days
(B) 7 days
(C) 9 days
(D) 11 days
(E) 33 days

# CHAPTER

# *60*
# Oxygen Extraction Ratio (O₂ER)

## NOTES

Oxygen extraction ratio ($O_2ER$) is also known as the oxygen utilization ratio or oxygen coefficient ratio. In the $O_2ER$ equation, $C_aO_2$ represents the total amount of oxygen available for peripheral tissue utilization, and $C_aO_2 - C_{\bar{v}}O_2$ reflects the amount of oxygen extracted or consumed by the peripheral tissues.

The $O_2ER$ provides a useful indication of a patient's oxygen transport status. Factors that cause a low $C_aO_2$ or a high $C(a-\bar{v})O_2$ lead to a high $O_2ER$ value. On the other hand, factors that contribute to a high $C_aO_2$ or a low $C(a-\bar{v})O_2$ result in a low $O_2ER$ value. Tables 8 and 9 summarize the major factors that affect the oxygen extraction ratio.

## EQUATION

$$O_2ER = \frac{C_aO_2 - C_{\bar{v}}O_2}{C_aO_2}$$

$O_2ER$ : Oxygen extraction ratio in %

$C_aO_2$ : Arterial oxygen content in vol%

$C_{\bar{v}}O_2$ : Mixed venous oxygen content in vol%

## NORMAL VALUE

20 to 28%

## EXAMPLE

Given: $C_aO_2 = 20$ vol%

$C_{\bar{v}}O_2 = 16$ vol%

What is the calculated oxygen extraction ratio ($O_2ER$)?

$$O_2ER = \frac{C_aO_2 - C_{\bar{v}}O_2}{C_aO_2}$$

$$= \frac{20 - 16}{20}$$

$$= \frac{4}{20}$$

$$= 0.2 \text{ or } 20\%$$

### TABLE 8.  Factors That Increase the O₂ER

Decreased cardiac output

Periods of increased oxygen consumption

   Exercise

   Seizures

   Shivering in postoperative patient

   Hyperthermia

Anemia

Decreased arterial oxygenation

From Des Jardins, T.R., *Cardiopulmonary Anatomy and Physiology: Essentials for Respiratory Care*, 3rd ed. Albany, NY: Delmar Publishers, 1998.

---

**TABLE 9.  Factors That Decrease the O$_2$ER**

Increased cardiac output

Peripheral shunting (e.g., sepsis, trauma)

Certain poisons (e.g., cyanide prevents cellular metabolism)

Hypothermia (slows cellular metabolism)

Increased hemoglobin concentration

Increased arterial oxygenation

---

From Des Jardins, T.R., *Cardiopulmonary Anatomy and Physiology: Essentials for Respiratory Care,* 3rd ed. Albany, NY: Delmar Publishers, 1998.

---

**EXERCISE**

What is the calculated oxygen extraction ratio (O$_2$ER) for a patient with the following oxygen contents:

$C_aO_2 = 19$ vol%

$C_{\bar{v}}O_2 = 16$ vol%

[Answer: O$_2$ER = 15.8%]

**REFERENCE**

Des Jardins

**SEE**

*Appendix D: Oxygen Transport Normal Ranges.*

## Self-Assessment Questions

60a. Given: $C_aO_2 = 21$ vol%, $C_{\bar{v}}O_2 = 16.5$ vol%. Calculate the oxygen extraction ratio (O$_2$ER).

(A) 4.5%

(B) 16.5%

(C) 21%

(D) 79%

(E) 100%

60b. For a patient with these oxygen contents: $C_aO_2 = 20.4$ vol%, $C_{\bar{v}}O_2 = 15.6$ vol%, what is the calculated oxygen extraction ratio (O$_2$ER)?

(A) 4.8%

(B) 15.6%

(C) 20.4%

(D) 23.5%

(E) 100%

60c. Which of the following pairs of oxygen content measurements has the highest oxygen extraction ratio?

| | $C_aO_2$ (vol%) | $C_{\bar{v}}O_2$ (vol%) |
|---|---|---|
| (A) | 19 | 15 |
| (B) | 19 | 16 |
| (C) | 20 | 16 |
| (D) | 20 | 17 |
| (E) | 21 | 16 |

60d. Which of the following pairs of oxygen content measurements has the lowest oxygen extraction ratio?

| | $C_aO_2$ (vol%) | $C_{\bar{v}}O_2$ (vol%) |
|---|---|---|
| (A) | 18.5 | 13.8 |
| (B) | 18.5 | 14.2 |
| (C) | 19.3 | 14.2 |
| (D) | 19.3 | 15.5 |
| (E) | 20.1 | 15.5 |

CHAPTER

# 61
# Partial Pressure of a Dry Gas

## NOTES

Dalton's law states that the partial pressures of all gases in a gas mixture equal the total pressure exerted by the gas mixture. Therefore, the partial pressure of a gas can be determined by multiplying the barometric pressure ($P_B$) and the percentage of the gas in the mixture ($\%_g$).

At high altitude, the $P_B$ decreases, and consequently the partial pressures of all gases also decrease. For example, at an altitude of 26,000 ft above sea level ($P_B = 270$ mm Hg), $PO_2 = 270$ mmHg $\times$ 0.21 = 56.7 mm Hg.) On the other hand, hyperbaric conditions (e.g., below sea level, hyperbaric chambers) increase the barometric pressure and partial pressures of all gases. At a depth of 66 ft below sea level ($P_B = 2280$ mm Hg), $PO_2 = 2280$ mm Hg $\times 0.21 = 478.8$ mm Hg.

Under normal clinical conditions, the barometric pressure varies very little. By increasing the percentage of a gas (oxygen concentration), a higher partial pressure of that gas may be achieved. This is the basis of oxygen therapy.

## EQUATION

$$P_g = P_B \times \%_g$$

$P_g$ : Partial pressure of a dry gas
$P_B$ : Barometric pressure in mm Hg
$\%_g$ : Percent of gas in the mixture

## EXAMPLE

What is the partial pressure of (a) nitrogen and (b) oxygen in an air sample at a barometric pressure of 720 mm Hg?
Since nitrogen occupies 78% of air:
A. $PN_2 = P_B \times \%N_2$
$= 720 \times 78\%$
$= 561.6$ mm Hg
Since oxygen occupies 21% of air:
B. $PO_2 = P_B \times \%0_2$
$= 720 \times 21\%$
$= 151.2$ mm Hg

## EXERCISE

Calculate the partial pressure of oxygen in a dry air sample at 40,000 ft above sea level ($P_B = 141$ mm Hg). ($F_IO_2$ at 40,000 ft above sea level = 21%.)

[Answer: $PO_2 = 29.6$ mm Hg]

## REFERENCE

Scanlan

## SEE

*Alveolar Oxygen Tension ($P_AO_2$); Dalton's Law of Partial Pressure; Appendix L: Barometric Pressures at Selected Altitudes.*

# Self-Assessment Questions

61a.  At sea level ($P_B$ = 760 mm Hg), what is the partial pressure of oxygen in a dry, ambient air sample?

(A) 80 mm Hg

(B) 100 mm Hg

(C) 115 mm Hg

(D) 126 mm Hg

(E) 159 mm Hg

61b.  At 33 ft below sea level ($P_B$ = 1520 mm Hg), what is the partial pressure of oxygen of a diver's inspired air?

(A) 190 mm Hg

(B) 200 mm Hg

(C) 230 mm Hg

(D) 252 mm Hg

(E) 319 mm Hg

61c.  Calculate the partial pressure of oxygen in a dry air sample at 10,000 ft above sea level ($P_B$ = 523 mm Hg).

(A) 80 mm Hg

(B) 94 mm Hg

(C) 110 mm Hg

(D) 122 mm Hg

(E) 218 mm Hg

61d.  Since carbon dioxide makes up 0.03% of ambient air, calculate its partial pressure in a dry air sample at sea level ($P_B$ = 760 mm Hg).

(A) 0.23 mm Hg

(B) 2.28 mm Hg

(C) 22.8 mm Hg

(D) 228 mm Hg

(E) 300 mm Hg

# CHAPTER

# *62*
## *P*CO2 to H2CO3

### NOTES

Carbonic acid ($H_2CO_3$) concentration is represented by the solubility coefficient (0.03) times the partial pressure of arterial carbon dioxide ($P_aCO_2$).

$H_2CO_3$ is an important factor in acid-base balance because of its role in determining the blood pH. Being the denominator of the Henderson-Hasselbalch equation, $H_2CO_3$ ($P_aCO_2$) is inversely related to the pH. In other words, a high $H_2CO_3$ ($P_aCO_2$) level with normal $HCO_3^-$ results in a low pH (acidosis). A low $H_2CO_3$ ($P_aCO_2$) level with normal $HCO_3^-$ results in a high pH (alkalosis).

Note also that the conversion factor used for $P_aCO_2$ to $H_2CO_3$ is 0.03 and that for $PO_2$ to oxygen content is 0.003. These two factors are quite similar, and they should be used with care.

### EQUATION

$$H_2CO_3 = P_aCO_2 \times 0.03$$

$H_2CO_3$:  Carbonate acid in mEq/L
$P_aCO_2$ :  Arterial carbon dioxide tension in mm Hg

### NORMAL VALUE

1.05 to 1.35 mEq/L

### EXAMPLE

Given: $P_aCO_2 = 40$ mm Hg
What is the calculated carbonic acid level?
$$\begin{aligned} H_2CO_3 &= P_aCO_2 \times 0.03 \\ &= 40 \times 0.03 \\ &= 1.2 \text{ mEq/L} \end{aligned}$$

### EXERCISE

Given: $P_aCO_2 = 50$ mm Hg
Calculate the $H_2CO_3$ level.

[Answer: $H_2CO_3 = 1.5$ mEq/L]

### REFERENCE

Shapiro (1)

### SEE

*pH (Henderson-Hasselbalch).*

# Self-Assessment Questions

62a. The amount of carbonic acid can be determined by using the equation:

(A) $0.003 \times P_aCO_2$

(B) $0.03 \times P_aCO_2$

(C) $0.3 \times P_aCO_2$

(D) $pK + \log \dfrac{HCO_3^-}{H_2CO_3}$

(E) $6.1 + \log \dfrac{HCO_3^-}{0.003 \times P_aCO_2}$

62b. Based on the pH equation, a $P_aCO_2$ of 50 mm Hg equals _____ mEq/L of carbonic acid.

(A) 1.5

(B) 1.2

(C) 1.0

(D) 0.5

(E) 0.03

62c. A blood gas measurement shows that the $P_aCO_2$ is 30 mm Hg. What is the calculated carbonic acid level?

(A) 0.15 mEq/L

(B) 1.5 mEq/L

(C) 15 mEq/L

(D) 0.9 mEq/L

(E) 9 mEq/L

62d. Which of the following $P_aCO_2$ values corresponds with a carbonic acid level of 1.2 mEq/L?

(A) 20 mm Hg

(B) 30 mm Hg

(C) 40 mm Hg

(D) 50 mm Hg

(E) 60 mm Hg

# CHAPTER

# 63
# pH (Henderson-Hasselbalch)

*NOTES*

The pH value is directly related to the bicarbonate ($HCO_3^-$) level, and it is inversely related to the carbonic acid ($H_2CO_3$) or the carbon dioxide tension ($PCO_2$) level.

Providing there is no compensation, the pH will be greater than 7.40 with an increase of $HCO_3^-$ (metabolic alkalosis) or a decrease of $PCO_2$ (respiratory alkalosis). In other words, if the $HCO_3^-$ : $H_2CO_3$ ratio is *greater than 20:1*, the pH will be *higher than 7.40.*

On the other hand, the pH will be less than 7.40 with a decrease of $HCO_3^-$ (metabolic acidosis) or an increase of $PCO_2$ (respiratory acidosis). In other words, if the $HCO_3^-$: $H_2CO_3$ ratio is *less than 20:1*, the pH will be *lower than 7.40.*

It is essential to note that the pH will be 7.40 as long as the $HCO_3^-$:$H_2CO_3$ ratio is 20:1. The Example and Exercise 1 illustrate this compensatory effect even though the $HCO_3^-$ and $PCO_2$ values are quite different in these two cases.

**EQUATION 1**

$$pH = 6.1 + \log\left[\frac{HCO_3^-}{H_2CO_3}\right]$$

**EQUATION 2**

$$pH = 6.1 + \log\left[\frac{HCO_3^-}{PCO_2 \times 0.03}\right]$$

pH : Puissance hydrogen, negative logarithm of $H^+$ ion concentration

$HCO_3^-$: Serum bicarbonate concentration in mEq/L

$H_2CO_3$: Carbonate acid in mEq/L

$PCO_2$ : Carbon dioxide tension in mm Hg

**NORMAL VALUE**

Arterial pH     = 7.40 (7.35 to 7.45)
Mixed venous pH = 7.36

**EXAMPLE**

Given: $H_2CO_3^-$:   24 mEq/L
        $PCO_2$   :   40 mm Hg
Calculate the pH.

$$pH = 6.1 + \log\left[\frac{HCO_3^-}{PCO_2 \times 0.03}\right]$$

$$= 6.1 + \log\left[\frac{24}{40 \times 0.03}\right]$$

$$= 6.1 + \log\left[\frac{24}{1.2}\right]$$

$$= 6.1 + \log 20$$

(From the common logarithms of numbers in Appendix M, log 20 = 1.301.)

$$pH = 6.1 + 1.301$$

$$= 7.401 \text{ or } 7.40$$

**EXERCISE 1**

Given: $HCO_3^- = 30\,mEq/L$

$PCO_2 = 50\,mm\,Hg$

$\log 20 = 1.301$

Calculate the pH.

[Answer: pH = 7.401 or 7.40]

**EXERCISE 2**

Given: $HCO_3^- = 16\,mEq/L$

$PCO_2 = 32\,mm\,Hg$

Use the Henderson-Hasselbalch equation and common logarithms of numbers in Appendix M to calculate the pH.

[Answer: pH = 7.32 since log 16.67 = 1.222]

**REFERENCES**

Shapiro (1); Wojciechowski

**SEE**

*Appendix M: Using the Logarithm Table.*

## Self-Assessment Questions

63a. When the ratio of bicarbonate to carbonic acid in blood is 20:1, the pH will be

(A) 6.80

(B) 7.20

(C) 7.40

(D) 7.60

(E) 7.80

63b. The pH is normal (7.40) when the bicarbonate to carbonic acid ratio is

(A) 20 : 1

(B) 24 : 1

(C) 1 : 20

(D) 1 : 24

(E) 1 : 26

63c. Given: $HCO_3^- = 30\,mEq/L$, $PCO_2 = 50\,mm\,Hg$. The calculated pH is about

(A) 7.20

(B) 7.25

(C) 7.35

(D) 7.40

(E) 7.45

63d. At a pH of 7.50, the ratio of bicarbonate to carbonic acid in blood is about

(A) 5:1

(B) 10:1

(C) 14:1

(D) 20:1

(E) 26:1

63e. From the logarithm table in Appendix M, find the value of log 20.

(A) 0.30

(B) 3.00

(C) 30.0

(D) 1.30

(E) 13.0

63f. From the logarithm table in Appendix M, find the value of log 16.

(A) 0.3

(B) 1.2

(C) 2.04

(D) 3

(E) 20.4

63g. Given: $HCO_3^- = 34$ mEq/L, $PCO_2 = 65$ mm Hg. Which of the following is used to calculate the pH? What is the calculated pH?

(A) $6.1 + \log 17.4$; 7.34

(B) $6.1 + \log 19.1$; 7.38

(C) $6.1 + \log 20.1$; 7.40

(D) $\log 19.1$; 7.38

(E) $\log 20.1$; 7.40

63h. Use the logarithm table in Appendix M to calculate the pH if the $HCO_3$- level is 16 mEq/L and $PCO_2 = 60$ mm Hg. Is the pH normal or abnormal?

(A) 7.05; normal

(B) 7.05; abnormal

(C) 7.11; normal

(D) 7.11; abnormal

(E) 7.23; abnormal

63i. Which of the following is *incorrect* with regard to the pH (Henderson-Hasselbalch) equation?

(A) The pH is directly related to the $HCO_3^-$ level.

(B) The pH is inversely related to the $PCO_2$ level.

(C) The pH will be 7.40 if the $HCO_3^-$ to $H_2CO_3$ ratio is 20:1.

(D) The pH will be less than 7.40 if the $HCO_3^-$ to $H_2CO_3$ ratio is less than 20:1.

(E) The pH will be less than 7.40 if the $HCO_3^-$ to $PCO_2$ ratio is less than 20:1.

# CHAPTER

# *64*
## Poiseuille's Law

**EQUATION**

$$\dot{V} = \frac{\Delta P r^4 \pi}{\mu l 8}$$

$\dot{V}$   :   Flow

$\Delta P$   :   Driving pressure

$r$   :   Radius of airway

$\dfrac{\pi}{8}$   :   Constant for equation

$\mu$   :   Viscosity of gas

$l$   :   Length of airway

Under clinical conditions where viscosity of gas ($\mu$), length of airway ($l$) and $\pi/8$ remain stable and unchanged, they may be deleted in order to look at the relationship among the remaining variables of the equation. The abbreviated form of Poiseuille's law is as follows:

$$\Delta P = \frac{\dot{V}}{r^4}$$

This equation shows that when the radius of the airway ($r$) decreases by half, the driving pressure ($\Delta P$) must increase 16 times to maintain the same flow. In other words, bronchoconstriction (decrease in $r$) can cause a tremendously large increase in the work of breathing (increase in $\Delta P$). If the work of breathing cannot keep up with the bronchoconstriction, air flow ($\dot{V}$) will be decreased.

In pulmonary function testing, reduction in flow rate measurements is generally indicative of bronchoconstriction.

**REFERENCE**    White

## Self-Assessment Questions

64a. Which of the following is the simplified form of Poiseuille's law describing the relationship between work of breathing and radius of airway?

(A) $\Delta P = \dot{V} \times r^2$

(B) $\Delta P = \dfrac{\dot{V}}{r^2}$

(C) $\Delta P = \dot{V} \times r^4$

(D) $\Delta P = \dfrac{\dot{V}}{r^4}$

(E) $\Delta P = \dfrac{\dot{V}}{r^{16}}$

64b. _____ shows that the size of the airway is directly related to the gas flow and inversely related to the work of breathing.

(A) Henry's law

(B) Law of LaPlace

(C) Poiseuille's law

(D) Law of Continuity

(E) Dalton's law

64c. Poiseuille's law shows that when the radius of the airway ($r$) decreases by half, the driving pressure ($\Delta P$) must increase _____ times to maintain the same flow rate.

(A) 2

(B) 4

(C) 6

(D) 12

(E) 16

64d. Bronchoconstriction can cause an increase in the work of breathing because of the changes in the _____ of the airway.

(A) cilia

(B) mucosa

(C) radius

(D) length

(E) mucus glands

# CHAPTER

# 65

# Predicted $P_aO_2$ Based on Age

*NOTES*

This equation is used to estimate the $P_aO_2$ value of a healthy person breathing room air. The predicted $P_aO_2$ decreases with age.

If the patient is in a semi-Fowler position, use the $P_aO_2$ (seated) equation.

**EQUATION 1**   $P_aO_2 \text{ (supine)} = 103.5 - (0.42 \times \text{Age})$

**EQUATION 2**   $P_aO_2 \text{ (seated)} = 104.2 - (0.27 \times \text{Age})$

| | | |
|---|---|---|
| $P_aO_2$ (supine) | : | Predicted $P_aO_2$ (mm Hg) in a supine position |
| $P_aO_2$ (seated) | : | Predicted $P_aO_2$ (mm Hg) in a seated position |
| Age | : | Patient's age in years |

**EXAMPLE**   What is the predicted $P_aO_2$ of a 60-year-old patient who is breathing spontaneously in a supine position?

$$
\begin{aligned}
P_aO_2 \text{ (supine)} &= 103.5 - (0.42 \times \text{Age}) \\
&= 103.5 - (0.42 \times 60) \\
&= 103.5 - 25.2 \\
&= 78.3 \text{ or } 78 \text{ mm Hg}
\end{aligned}
$$

**EXERCISE**   Calculate the predicted $P_aO_2$ for a healthy 40-year-old patient who is spontaneously breathing room air in a sitting position.

[Answer: $P_aO_2$ (seated) = 93.4 or 93 mm Hg]

**REFERENCE**   Krider

**SEE**   *$F_IO_2$ Needed for a Desired $P_aO_2$.*

## Self-Assessment Questions

65a.  Given the equation to calculate the predicted $PO_2$ in a supine position: $PO_2$ (supine) = 103.5 – (0.42 × Age). What is the predicted $PO_2$ of a 50-year-old patient who is breathing spontaneously in a supine position?

(A) 73 mm Hg

(B)  78 mm Hg

(C)  83 mm Hg

(D) 87 mm Hg

(E)  90 mm Hg

65b.  Use the equation below to calculate the predicted $PO_2$ for a 50-year-old patient who is breathing room air spontaneously in a sitting position.
$PO_2$ (seated) = 104.2 – (0.27 × Age)

(A) 71 mm Hg

(B)  77 mm Hg

(C)  80 mm Hg

(D) 86 mm Hg

(E)  91 mm Hg

# CHAPTER

# *66*
# Relative Humidity

## NOTES

Relative humidity is usually measured by hygrometers, thus eliminating the need for extracting and measuring the humidity content of the air samples. The Examples illustrate how humidity content and capacity are related to the relative humidity.

Since the capacity is directly related to the temperature, a higher temperature causes the capacity to increase. If the content remains constant, a higher temperature or capacity ensures a *lower* relative humidity; the converse is also true.

Heated aerosol therapy provides two components to respiratory care. First, the heat increases the capacity of the gas mixture to carry humidity. Second, the aerosol increases the content (actual humidity) of the inspired gas, thus lowering the humidity deficit.

## EQUATION

$$RH = \frac{Content}{Capacity}$$

RH  : Relative humidity in %

Content : Humidity content of a volume of gas in mg / L or mm Hg; also known as actual or absolute humidity

Capacity : Humidity capacity or maximum amount of water that air can hold at a given temperature, in mg / L or mm Hg; also known as maximum absolute humidity.

## NORMAL VALUE

The relative humidity is directly proportional to the content.

## EXAMPLE 1

What is the relative humidity if the content of an air sample is 12 mg / L and its capacity is 18 mg / L?

$$RH = \frac{Content}{Capacity}$$

$$= \frac{12}{18}$$

$$= 0.67 \text{ or } 67\%$$

## EXAMPLE 2

Calculate the relative humidity if the content of an air sample is 16 mg / L and its capacity is 18 mg / L.

$$RH = \frac{Content}{Capacity}$$

$$= \frac{16}{18}$$

$$= 0.89 \text{ or } 89\%$$

## EXAMPLE 2

Calculate the relative humidity if the content of an air sample is 16 mg / L and its capacity is 20 mg / L.

$$RH = \frac{Content}{Capacity}$$

$$= \frac{16}{20}$$

$$= 0.8 \text{ or } 80\%$$

**EXERCISE 1**  An air sample has a humidity content of 15 mg/L and a capacity of 26 mg/L. What is the calculated relative humidity of this air sample?

[Answer: RH = 0.577 or 58%]

**EXERCISE 2**  Calculate the relative humidity of an air sample if the humidity content and capacity are 25 mg/L and 43 mg/L, respectively.

[Answer: RH = 0.581 or 58%]

**REFERENCES**  Scanlan; White

**SEE**  *Humidity Deficit; Appendix E: Factors for Converting Gas Volumes from ATPS to BTPS; Appendix I: Humidity Capacity of Saturated Gas at Selected Temperatures.*

## Self-Assessment Questions

66a.  What is the relative humidity if the humidity content of an air sample is 12 mg/L and the humidity capacity is 24 mg/L?

(A) 20%

(B) 40%

(C) 50%

(D) 60%

(E) 200%

66b.  Calculate the relative humidity of an air sample if its humidity content is 14 mg/L and the humidity capacity is 19 mg/L.

(A) 33%

(B) 74%

(C) 80%

(D) 85%

(E) 136%

66c. An air sample has a humidity content of 23 mg/L and a capacity of 26 mg/L at 100% saturation. Calculate the relative humidity of this sample.

(A) 32%

(B) 64%

(C) 78%

(D) 88%

(E) 113%

# 67
# Reynolds' Number

*NOTE*

Osborne Reynolds (1842–1912), an English scientist, developed a dimensionless number (ratio) to describe the dynamics of fluid and air flows.

**EQUATION**

$$R_N = \frac{v \times D \times d}{\mu}$$

$R_N$ : Reynolds number
$v$ : Velocity of fluid
$D$ : Fluid density
$d$ : Diameter of tube
$\mu$ : Viscosity of fluid

When the Reynolds number is less than 2000, it reflects laminar flow; when over 2000 it reflects turbulent flow. In actuality, values between 2000 and 4000 provide a mixed or transitional pattern (laminar and turbulent), but most respiratory care references refer to values within this range as turbulent flow. The gas flow characteristics of this equation can be applied to respiratory care. An increase in gas flow rate ($v$) or gas density ($D$) will increase the Reynolds number, thus making a turbulent flow more likely. Oxygen/helium mixture has been used to reduce the gas density so as to enhance gas flow and diffusion of oxygen.

An increase in airway size ($d$) does not increase the Reynolds number because the resulting lower flow rate ($v$) due to larger airway diameter tends to offset any significant change in the Reynolds number.

**REFERENCES**  Barnes; Pierson; Scanlan; Wojciechowski

## Self-Assessment Questions

67a.  Reynolds' number is used to describe the characteristic of

(A) fluid and air flow

(B) gas density

(C) lung elasticity

(D) lung compliance

(E) acid-base balance

67b. Laminar flow is expected when the
  (A) gas passes beyond the nasal cavity
  (B) flow is greater than 4 L/min
  (C) flow is less than 4 L/min
  (D) Reynolds' number is greater than 4000
  (E) Reynolds' number is less than 2000

67c. Oxygen/helium mixtures have been used on patients with airway obstruction because these mixtures provide a(n) _____ of gas density and _____ gas flow and diffusion of oxygen.
  (A) increase; increase
  (B) decrease; decrease
  (C) increase; decrease
  (D) decrease; increase
  (E) no change; increase

67d. An increase in airway size _____ the Reynolds number because the resulting _____ flow rate ($\dot{V}$) offsets any significant change in Reynolds' number.
  (A) increases; higher
  (B) decreases; higher
  (C) increases; lower
  (D) decreases; lower
  (E) does not change; lower

CHAPTER

# *68*
# Shunt Equation ($Q_{sp}/\dot{Q}_T$): Classic Physiologic

**NOTES**

The shunt equation is used to calculate the portion of cardiac output not taking part in gas exchange—wasted perfusion. The classic physiologic shunt equation requires an arterial sample for $C_aO_2$ and a mixed venous sample for $C_{\bar{v}}O_2$.

A calculated shunt of less than 10% is considered normal in clinical settings. Shunt of 10 to 20% indicates mild intrapulmonary shunting, and shunt of 20 to 30% indicates significant intrapulmonary shunting. Greater than 30% of calculated shunt reflects critical and severe intrapulmonary shunting. $Q_{sp}/\dot{Q}_T$ is increased in the presence of one of the following categories of shunt-producing diseases: *Anatomic shunt* (e.g., congenital heart disease, intrapulmonary fistulas, vascular lung tumors); *capillary shunt* (e.g., atelectasis, alveolar fluid); *venous admixture* (e.g., hypoventilation, uneven distribution of ventilation, diffusion defects).

**EQUATION**

$$\frac{Q_{sp}}{\dot{Q}_T} = \frac{C_cO_2 - C_aO_2}{C_cO_2 - C_{\bar{v}}O_2}$$

$Q_{sp}/\dot{Q}_T$ : Physiologic shunt to total perfusion ratio in %

$C_cO_2$ : End-capillary oxygen content in vol%

$C_aO_2$ : Arterial oxygen content in vol%

$C_{\bar{v}}O_2$ : Mixed venous oxygen content in vol%

**NORMAL VALUE**

Less than 10%

**EXAMPLE**

Given: $C_cO_2$ = 20.4 vol%

$\quad\quad C_aO_2$ = 19.8 vol%

$\quad\quad C_{\bar{v}}O_2$ = 13.4 vol%

$$Q_{sp}/\dot{Q}_T = \frac{C_cO_2 - C_aO_2}{C_cO_2 - C_{\bar{v}}O_2}$$

$$= \frac{20.4 - 19.8}{20.4 - 13.4}$$

$$= \frac{0.6}{7}$$

$$= 0.086 \text{ or } 8.6\%$$

**EXERCISE**

Given: $C_cO_2$ = 20.6 vol%

$\quad\quad C_aO_2$ = 17.2 vol%

$\quad\quad C_{\bar{v}}O_2$ = 10.6 vol%

Calculate the $Q_{sp}/\dot{Q}_T$. Is it normal or abnormal?

[Answer: $Q_{sp}/\dot{Q}_T$ = 34%. Severe intrapulmonary shunting.]

**REFERENCES** Shapiro (1); Malley

**SEE** *Oxygen Content: End-capillary ($C_cO_2$) for calculation of $C_cO_2$. Shunt Equation ($Qsp/\dot{Q}_T$): Estimated; Appendix D: Oxygen Transport Normal Ranges.*

## Self-Assessment Questions

68a. Normal cardiopulmonary function usually provides a calculated shunt of

   (A) 10% or less

   (B) 20% or less

   (C) 30% or less

   (D) 40% or less

   (E) 60% or less

68b. The classic physiologic shunt equation is represented by

   (A) $(C_aO_2 - C_{\bar{v}}O_2) \times (C_cO_2 - C_aO_2)$

   (B) $\dfrac{C_aO_2 - C_{\bar{v}}O_2}{C_cO_2 - C_aO_2}$

   (C) $\dfrac{C_cO_2 - C_{\bar{v}}O_2}{C_cO_2 - C_aO_2}$

   (D) $(C_cO_2 - C_aO_2) \times (C_cO_2 - C_{\bar{v}}O_2)$

   (E) $\dfrac{C_cO_2 - C_aO_2}{C_cO_2 - C_{\bar{v}}O_2}$

68c. The ($C_cO_2 - C_aO_2$) portion of the classic physiologic shunt equation represents

   (A) oxygen consumption

   (B) shunted perfusion

   (C) total perfusion

   (D) oxygen content

   (E) oxygen tension

68d. Given: $C_cO_2$ = 21.1 vol%, $C_aO_2$ = 18.8 vol%, $C_{\bar{v}}O_2$ = 14.4 vol%. Calculate the percent shunt using the classic physiologic shunt equation. Is it normal or abnormal?

   (A) 10%; normal

   (B) 34%; abnormal

   (C) 34%; normal

   (D) 66%; abnormal

   (E) 66%; normal

68e. Given: $C_cO_2$ = 20.5 vol%, $C_aO_2$ = 20.1 vol%, $C_{\bar{v}}O_2$ = 13.8 vol%. Calculate the percent shunt using the classic physiologic shunt equation. Is it normal or abnormal?

   (A) 6%; normal

(B) 6%; abnormal

(C) 12%; normal

(D) 12%; abnormal

(E) 20%; normal

68f. A patient in the intensive care unit has the following oxygen content measurements: $C_aO_2$ = 19.7 vol%, $C_{\bar{v}}O_2$ = 13.6 vol%. If the calculated $C_cO_2$ is 20.8 vol%, what is the percent shunt based on the classic physiologic shunt equation? Is the calculated shunt normal, mild, moderate, or severe for this patient?

(A) 10%; normal shunt

(B) 10%; mild shunt

(C) 15%; mild shunt

(D) 15%; moderate shunt

(E) 20%; severe shunt

68g. A patient who is diagnosed with adult respiratory distress syndrome has a $C_cO_2$ of 21 vol%, $C_aO_2$ of 18.2 vol%, and $C_{\bar{v}}O_2$ of 14 vol%. Use the classic physiologic shunt equation to calculate the shunt percent. Is it consistent with the diagnosis?

(A) 20%; normal, inconsistent with diagnosis

(B) 20%; mild shunt, inconsistent with diagnosis

(C) 30%; mild shunt, inconsistent with diagnosis

(D) 40%; moderate shunt, consistent with diagnosis

(E) 40%; severe shunt, consistent with diagnosis

68h. Which of the following sets of oxygen content measurement has the *highest* calculated physiologic shunt?

| | $C_cO_2$ | $C_aO_2$ | $C_{\bar{v}}O_2$ (vol%) |
|---|---|---|---|
| (A) | 20 | 19 | 15 |
| (B) | 19 | 17 | 14 |
| (C) | 21 | 20 | 16 |
| (D) | 18 | 17 | 13 |
| (E) | 17 | 16 | 12 |

68i. Which of the following sets of oxygen content measurement has the *lowest* calculated physiologic shunt?

| | $C_cO_2$ | $C_aO_2$ | $C_{\bar{v}}O_2$ (vol%) |
|---|---|---|---|
| (A) | 20.8 | 18.7 | 14.3 |
| (B) | 18.7 | 16.9 | 13.2 |
| (C) | 20.1 | 19.0 | 14.6 |
| (D) | 18.4 | 17.2 | 13.5 |
| (E) | 17.3 | 16.0 | 13.3 |

68j. Which of the following sets of oxygen content measurement represents *normal* physiologic shunt?

| | $C_cO_2$ | $C_aO_2$ | $C_{\bar{v}}O_2$ (vol%) |
|---|---|---|---|
| (A) | 19.8 | 19.0 | 14.3 |
| (B) | 20.3 | 18.2 | 13.6 |
| (C) | 17.1 | 16.8 | 12.9 |
| (D) | 18.3 | 17.5 | 13.8 |
| (E) | 18.6 | 16.7 | 12.9 |

68k. A patient has a series of physiologic shunts measured; they are listed as follows. Which of the following sets of oxygen content measurement represents a severe physiologic shunt?

|  | $C_cO_2$ | $C_aO_2$ | $C_{\bar{v}}O_2$ (vol%) |
|---|---|---|---|
| (A) | 20.3 | 17.8 | 13.6 |
| (B) | 19.6 | 19.0 | 14.7 |
| (C) | 19.1 | 17.7 | 13.5 |
| (D) | 18.5 | 17.9 | 13.8 |
| (E) | 19.0 | 17.6 | 13.1 |

# 69
# Shunt Equation ($Q_{sp}/\dot{Q}_T$): Estimated

## NOTES

The estimated shunt equation does not require a mixed venous blood sample. It is less accurate than the classic physiologic shunt equation. In normal subjects, 5 vol% may be used as the estimated arterial–mixed venous oxygen content difference [$C(a-\bar{v})O_2$]. In critically ill patients, 3.5 vol% may be used since it is common for such patients to have a lower $C(a-\bar{v})O_2$ due to increased cardiac output or decreased oxygen consumption (extraction).

A calculated shunt of less than 10% is considered normal in clinical settings. Shunt of 10 to 20% indicates mild intrapulmonary shunting, and shunt of 20 to 30% is indicative of significant intrapulmonary shunting. Greater than 30% of calculated shunt reflects critical and severe intrapulmonary shunting.

$Q_{sp}/\dot{Q}_T$ is increased in the presence of one of the following categories of shunt-producing disease: *Anatomic shunt* (e.g., congenital heart disease, intrapulmonary fistulas, vascular lung tumors); *capillary shunt* (e.g., atelectasis, alveolar fluid); *venous admixture* (e.g., hypoventilation, uneven distribution of ventilation, diffusion defects).

## EQUATION 1

For individuals who are breathing spontaneously with or without CPAP:

$$\frac{Q_{sp}}{\dot{Q}_T} = \frac{C_cO_2 - C_aO_2}{5 + (C_cO_2 - C_aO_2)}$$

## EQUATION 2

For critically ill patients who are receiving mechanical ventilation with or without PEEP:

$$\frac{Q_{sp}}{\dot{Q}_T} = \frac{C_cO_2 - C_aO_2}{3.5 + (C_cO_2 - C_aO_2)}$$

$Q_{sp}/\dot{Q}_T$ : Physiologic shunt to total perfusion ratio in %
$C_cO_2$ : End-capillary oxygen content in vol%
$C_aO_2$ : Arterial oxygen content in vol%

## NORMAL VALUE

Less than 10%

## EXAMPLE 1

Given: A patient on CPAP of 5 cmH₂O
$C_cO_2$ = 20.4 vol%
$C_aO_2$ = 19.8 vol%
Use 5 vol% as the estimated $C(a-\bar{v})O_2$ and calculate $Q_{sp}/\dot{Q}_T$.

$$\frac{Q_{sp}}{\dot{Q}_T} = \frac{C_cO_2 - C_aO_2}{5 + (C_cO_2 - C_aO_2)}$$

$$= \frac{20.4 - 19.8}{5 + (20.4 - 19.8)}$$

$$= \frac{0.6}{5 + 0.6}$$

$$= \frac{0.6}{5.6}$$

$$= 0.107 \text{ or } 10.7\%$$

**EXAMPLE 2**

Given: A patient on mechanical ventilation

$C_cO_2$  =  20.4 vol%

$C_aO_2$  =  19.8 vol%

Use 3.5 vol% as the estimated $C(a-\bar{v})O_2$ and calculate $Q_{sp}/\dot{Q}_T$.

$$\frac{Q_{sp}}{\dot{Q}_T} = \frac{C_cO_2 - C_aO_2}{3.5 + (C_cO_2 - C_aO_2)}$$

$$= \frac{20.4 - 19.8}{3.5 + (20.4 - 19.8)}$$

$$= \frac{0.6}{3.5 + 0.6}$$

$$= \frac{0.6}{4.1}$$

$$= 0.146 \text{ or } 14.6\%$$

**EXERCISE 1**

Given: $C_cO_2$   =  20.6 vol%

$C_aO_2$  =  19.8 vol%

Use $C(a-\bar{v})O_2$ of 5 vol% and calculate the estimated $Q_{sp}/\dot{Q}_T$ of a patient. Is it normal?

[Answer: $Q_{sp}/\dot{Q}_T = 0.138$ or 13.8%. Abnormal, mild shunt.]

**EXERCISE 2**

Given the oxygen contents of a critically ill patient who is receiving mechanical ventilation:

$C_cO_2$  =  20.6 vol%

$C_aO_2$  =  17.2 vol%

Use $C(a-\bar{v})O_2$ of 3.5 vol% and calculate the estimated $Q_{sp}/\dot{Q}_T$ of this critically ill patient. Is it normal?

[Answer: $Q_{sp}/\dot{Q}_T = 0.49$ or 49%. Abnormal, severe shunt.]

**REFERENCES**

Shapiro (1); Malley

**SEE**

*Shunt Equation ($Q_{sp}/\dot{Q}_T$): Classic Physiologic; Appendix D: Oxygen Transport Normal Ranges.*

## Self-Assessment Questions

69a.  All of the following are true with regard to the estimated shunt equation with the *exception* of

(A)  It does not require placement of a pulmonary artery catheter.

(B)  It does not require a mixed venous sample.

(C)  It does not require a $C_{\bar{v}}O_2$ value.

(D)  Its accuracy is the same as that of the classic physiologic shunt equation.

(E)  It requires only an arterial blood sample.

69b.  The estimated physiologic shunt equation for individuals not receiving mechanical ventilation is:

(A)  $\dfrac{C_cO_2 - C_aO_2}{C_cO_2 - C_{\bar{v}}O_2}$

(B)  $(C_cO_2 - C_aO_2) \times (5 + C_cO_2 - C_aO_2)$

(C)  $\dfrac{C_cO_2 - C_aO_2}{5 + C_cO_2 - C_aO_2}$

(D)  $(C_aO_2 - C_{\bar{v}}O_2) \times (5 + C_cO_2 - C_aO_2)$

(E)  $\dfrac{C_aO_2 - C_{\bar{v}}O_2}{5 + C_cO_2 - C_aO_2}$

69c.  Given: $C_cO_2 = 20.4$ vol%, $C_aO_2 = 19.7$ vol%. Calculate the estimated $\dfrac{Q_{sp}}{\dot{Q}_T}$. Is it normal? (Assume $C_aO_2 - C_{\bar{v}}O_2 = 5$ vol% for individuals not receiving mechanical ventilation)

(A)  12.3%; normal

(B)  12.3%; mild shunt

(C)  23.6%; normal

(D)  23.6%; moderate shunt

(E)  35.2%; severe shunt

69d.  A *critically ill* patient has a $C_aO_2$ of 14.5 vol%. If the calculated end-capillary oxygen content is 16.8 vol%, what is the estimated shunt for this patient? How severe is the shunt? (Assume $C_aO_2 - C_{\bar{v}}O_2 = 3.5$ vol% for critically ill patients.)

(A)  24.8%; mild shunt

(B)  24.8%; moderate shunt

(C)  39.6%; mild shunt

(D)  39.6%; moderate shunt

(E)  39.6%; severe shunt

69e.  Which of the following sets of values has the *highest* estimated shunt?

|     | $C_cO_2$ | $C_aO_2$ (vol%) |
| --- | --- | --- |
| (A) | 20 | 19 |
| (B) | 19 | 17 |
| (C) | 21 | 20 |
| (D) | 18 | 17 |
| (E) | 17 | 16 |

69f.  Which of the following sets of values has the *lowest* estimated shunt?

| | $C_cO_2$ | $C_aO_2$ (vol%) |
|---|---|---|
| (A) | 20.8 | 18.7 |
| (B) | 18.7 | 16.9 |
| (C) | 20.1 | 19.0 |
| (D) | 18.4 | 17.2 |
| (E) | 17.3 | 16.0 |

69g.  Which of the following sets of values represents a *normal* estimated shunt?

| | $C_cO_2$ | $C_aO_2$ (vol%) |
|---|---|---|
| (A) | 19.8 | 19.0 |
| (B) | 20.3 | 18.2 |
| (C) | 17.1 | 16.8 |
| (D) | 18.3 | 17.5 |
| (E) | 18.6 | 16.7 |

69h.  A patient's arterial oxygen contents are listed below. With the respective end-capillary oxygen content, which of the following sets of values shows a severe physiologic shunt?

| | $C_cO_2$ | $C_aO_2$ (vol%) |
|---|---|---|
| (A) | 20.3 | 17.8 |
| (B) | 19.6 | 19.0 |
| (C) | 19.1 | 17.7 |
| (D) | 18.5 | 17.9 |
| (E) | 19.0 | 17.6 |

69i.  The following values are obtained from a *critically ill* patient: $C_cO_2 = 20.5$ vol%, $C_aO_2 = 18.6$ vol%, $C_{\bar{v}}O_2 = 14.8$ vol%. Calculate the percent shunt using the classic physiologic shunt equation. Assuming $C_aO_2 - C_{\bar{v}}O_2 = 3.5$ vol%, calculate the estimated shunt.

(A)  classic 23.8%; estimated 34.6%

(B)  classic 33.3%; estimated 35.2%

(C)  classic 33.3%; estimated 36.5%

(D)  classic 34.1%; estimated 27.5%

(E)  classic 34.1%; estimated 36.5%

# *70*

# Shunt Equation: Modified

**EQUATION**

$$\frac{Q_s}{\dot{Q}_T} = \frac{(P_AO_2 - P_aO_2) \times 0.003}{(C_aO_2 - C_{\bar{v}}O_2) + (P_AO_2 - P_aO_2) \times 0.003}$$

$\dfrac{Q_s}{\dot{Q}_T}$ : Modified shunt in %

$P_AO_2$ : Alveolar oxygen tension in mm Hg

$P_aO_2$ : Arterial oxygen tension in mm Hg

$C_aO_2$ : Arterial oxygen content in vol%

$C_{\bar{v}}O_2$ : Mixed venous oxygen content in vol%

This equation is modified from the classic physiologic shunt equation in which $(P_AO_2 - P_aO_2) \times 0.003$ is used to substitute for $C_cO_2 - C_aO_2$. The equation requires an arterial $PO_2$ greater than 150 mm Hg. Since most patients do not achieve this level of $PO_2$, it has limited clinical application.

A further simplified equation, $P_AO_2 - P_aO_2$, consisting of only a portion of the modified shunt equation, has been used to estimate the degree of physiologic shunt. To increase the accuracy of this simplified equation, the $P_AO_2$ and $P_aO_2$ values are usually measured on an $F_IO_2$ of 100%.

**REFERENCE**

Barnes

**SEE**

*Shunt Equation: Classic Physiologic.*
*Alveolar–Arterial Oxygen Tension Gradient $P(A - a)O_2$.*

## Self-Assessment Questions

70a. In the modified shunt equation, $(P_AO_2 - P_aO_2) \times 0.003$ is used to substitute for _____ of the classic physiologic shunt equation.

(A) $C_cO_2 - C_aO_2$

(B) $C_aO_2 - C_{\bar{v}}O_2$

(C) $C_{\bar{v}}O_2 - C_aO_2$

(D) $C_cO_2 - C_{\bar{v}}O_2$

(E) $C_{\bar{v}}O_2 - C_cO_2$

70b. To be accurate, the modified shunt equation should have an arterial $PO_2$ greater than _____ mm Hg.

(A) 60

(B) 80

(C) 100

(D) 120

(E) 150

CHAPTER

# *71*

# Stroke Volume (*SV*) and Stroke Volume Index (*SVI*)

*NOTES*

The stroke volume (*SV*) measures the average cardiac output per one heartbeat. Its accuracy is dependent on the method and technique used in the cardiac output measurement (e.g., Fick's estimated method, dye-dilution, and thermodilution).

The *SV* is increased by drugs that raise cardiac contractility and during early stages of compensated septic shock. It is decreased by drugs that lower cardiac contractility and during late stages of decompensated septic shock.

The stroke volume index (*SVI*) is used to normalize stroke volume measurement among patients of varying body size. For instance, a 50-mL stroke volume may be normal for an average-sized person but low for a large person. The *SVI* will be able to distinguish this difference based on the body size. See Table 10 for factors that change *SV*, *SVI*, and other hemodynamic measurements.

**EQUATION 1**

$$SV = \frac{CO}{HR}$$

**EQUATION 2**

$$SVI = \frac{SV}{BSA}$$

$SV$ : Stroke volume in mL or L (or mL/beat)

$SVI$ : Stroke volume index in mL/m$^2$ (or mL/beat/m$^2$)

$CO$ : Cardiac output in L/min ($\dot{Q}_T$)

$HR$ : Heart rate/min

$BSA$: Body surface area in m$^2$

**NORMAL VALUES**

$SV$ : 40 to 80 mL

$SVI$ : 33 to 47 mL/m$^2$

**EXAMPLE**

Given: Cardiac output  = 4.0 L/min

Heart rate  = 100/min

Body surface area  = 1.5 m$^2$

Calculate the stroke volume and the stroke volume index.

$$SV = \frac{CO}{HR}$$

$$= \frac{4.0}{100}$$

$$= 0.04 \text{ L or } 40 \text{ mL}$$

$$SVI = \frac{SV}{BSA}$$

$$= \frac{40}{1.5}$$

$$= 26.7 \text{ mL/m}^2$$

**TABLE 10   Factors Increasing and Decreasing Stroke Volume (*SV*), Stroke Volume Index (*SVI*), Cardiac Output (*CO*), Cardiac Index (*CI*), Right Ventricular Stroke Work Index (*RVSWI*), and Left Ventricular Stroke Work Index (*LVSWI*)**

**INCREASES**
**Positive Inotrophic Drugs (Increased Contractility)**
Dobutamine (Dobutrex®)
Epinephrine (Adrenalin®)
Dopamine (Intropin®)
Isoproterenol (Isuprel®)
Digitalis
Amrinone (Inocor®)

**Abnormal Conditions**
Septic shock (early stages)
Hyperthermia
Hypervolemia
Decreased vascular resistance

**DECREASES**
**Negative Inotropic Drugs (Decreased Contractility)**
Propranolol (Inderal®)
Timolol (Blocadren®)
Metoprolol (Lopressor®)
Atenolol (Tenormin®)
Nadolol (Corgard®)

**Abnormal Conditions**
Septic shock (late stages)
Congestive heart failure
Hypovolemia
Pulmonary emboli
Increased vascular resistance
Myocardial infarction

**Hyperinflation of Lungs**
Mechanical ventilation
   Continuous Positive Airway Pressure (CPAP)
   Positive End-Expiratory Pressure (PEEP)

From Des Jardins, T.R., *Cardiopulmonary Anatomy and Physiology: Essentials for Respiratory Care*, 3rd ed. Albany, NY: Delmar Publishers, 1998.

**EXERCISE**

Given: Cardiac output    = 5.0 L/min
       Heart rate        = 80/min
       Body surface area = 1.2 m²

Calculate the stroke volume and the stroke volume index.

[Answer: *SV* = 62.5 mL; *SVI* = 52.1 mL/m²]

**REFERENCES**    Bustin; Des Jardins

**SEE**    *Cardiac Output CO: Fick's Estimated Method; Cardiac Index (CI); Appendix F: DuBois Body Surface Chart; Appendix G: Hemodynamic Normal Ranges.*

# Self-Assessment Questions

71a. The equation for calculating the stroke volume (*SV*) is

(A) Cardiac output × Heart rate

(B) $\dfrac{\text{Cardiac output}}{\text{Heart rate}}$

(C) $\dfrac{\text{Cardiac output × Heart rate}}{\text{Body surface area}}$

(D) $\dfrac{\text{Cardiac output / Heart rate}}{\text{Body surface area}}$

(E) $\dfrac{\text{Cardiac output}}{\text{Body surface area}}$

71b. The equation for calculating the stroke volume index (*SVI*) is

(A) Cardiac output × Heart rate

(B) $\dfrac{\text{Cardiac output}}{\text{Heart rate}}$

(C) $\dfrac{\text{Cardiac output × Heart rate}}{\text{Body surface area}}$

(D) $\dfrac{\text{Cardiac output / Heart rate}}{\text{Body surface area}}$

(E) $\dfrac{\text{Cardiac output}}{\text{Body surface area}}$

71c. Given: cardiac output = 4.5 L/min, heart rate = 110/min, body surface area = 1.3 m$^2$. Calculate the stroke volume (*SV*) and stroke volume index (*SVI*).

(A) $SV = 49.5$ mL; $SVI = 38.1$ mL/m$^2$

(B) $SV = 46.2$ mL; $SVI = 35.5$ mL/m$^2$

(C) $SV = 44.6$ mL; $SVI = 34.3$ mL/m$^2$

(D) $SV = 42.0$ mL; $SVI = 32.3$ mL/m$^2$

(E) $SV = 40.9$ mL; $SVI = 31.5$ mL/m$^2$

71d. A patient whose body surface area is about 1.1 m$^2$ has the following hemodynamic measurements: cardiac output = 5.9 L/min, heart rate = 120/min. Calculate the stroke volume (*SV*) and stroke volume index (*SVI*).

(A) $SV = 70.8$ mL; $SVI = 51.6$ mL/m$^2$

(B) $SV = 70.8$ mL; $SVI = 64.4$ mL/m$^2$

(C) $SV = 49.2$ mL; $SVI = 40.7$ mL/m$^2$

(D) $SV = 49.2$ mL; $SVI = 44.7$ mL/m$^2$

(E) $SV = 51.7$ mL; $SVI = 47.0$ mL/m$^2$

71e. Given the following stroke volume (*SV*) and body surface area (*BSA*) measurements, which set of values has the highest stroke volume index (*SVI*)?

|  | *SV* (mL) | *BSA* (m$^2$) |
|---|---|---|
| (A) | 60 | 1.4 |
| (B) | 55 | 1.2 |
| (C) | 58 | 2.0 |
| (D) | 63 | 1.7 |
| (E) | 66 | 1.8 |

# 72

# Stroke Work: Left Ventricular (*LVSW*) and Index (*LVSWI*)

## NOTES

Left ventricular stroke work (*LVSW*) reflects the work of the left heart in providing perfusion through the systemic circulation. *LVSW* is directly related to the systemic vascular resistance, myocardial mass, and the volume and viscosity of the blood. In addition, tachycardia, hypoxemia, and poor contractility of the heart may further increase the stroke work of the left heart.

The pulmonary capillary wedge pressure (*PCWP*) is used because it approximates the mean left atrial pressure or the left ventricle end-diastolic pressure.

The constant 0.0136 in the equation is used to convert mm Hg/mL to gram · meters (g · m).

The left ventricular stroke work index (*LVSWI*) is used to equalize the stroke work to a person's body size. In the example shown, an apparently low left ventricular stroke work may be normal for a small person after indexing. See Fig. 40 for the relationship between *LVSWI* and left ventricular preload (represented by *PCWP*). For example, when the *LVSWI* and *PCWP* readings are both low and meet in quadrant 1, hypovolemia may be present.

## EQUATION 1

$$LVSW = (BP_{\text{systolic}} - PCWP) \times SV \times 0.0136$$

## EQUATION 2

$$LVSWI = \frac{LVSW}{BSA}$$

| | | |
|---|---|---|
| *LVSW* | : | Left ventricular stroke work in g · m/beat |
| *LVSWI* | : | Left ventricular stroke work index in g · m/beat/m$^2$ |
| $BP_{\text{systolic}}$ | : | Systolic blood pressure in mm Hg |
| *PCWP* | : | Pulmonary capillary wedge pressure in mm Hg |
| *SV* | : | Stroke volume in mL |
| *BSA* | : | Body surface area in m$^2$ |

## NORMAL VALUES

$$LVSW = 60 \text{ to } 80 \text{ g} \cdot \text{m/beat}$$
$$LVSWI = 40 \text{ to } 60 \text{ g} \cdot \text{m/beat/m}^2$$

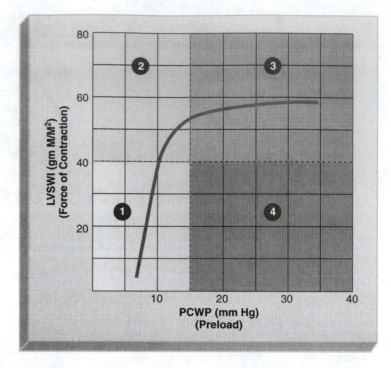

**Figure 40** *Frank-Starling curve. The Frank-Starling curve shows that the more the myocardial fiber is stretched as a result of the blood pressure that develops as blood returns to the chambers of the heart during diastole, the more the heart muscle will contract during systole. In addition, it will contract with greater force. The stretch produced within the myocardium at end-diastole is called preload. Clinically, it would be best to determine the preload of the left ventricle by measuring the end-diastolic pressure of the left ventricle or left atrium. However, since it is impractical to measure that at the patient's bedside, the best preload approximation of the left heart is the pulmonary capillary wedge pressure (PCWP). As shown in this illustration, the relationship of the PCWP (preload) to the left ventricular stroke work index (LVSWI) (force of contraction) may appear in four quadrants: (1) hypovolemia, (2) optimal function, (3) hypervolemia, and (4) cardiac failure.*

## EXAMPLE

Given: 
$$BP \quad = \quad 100/60 \text{ mm Hg}$$
$$PCWP \quad = \quad 20 \text{ mm Hg}$$
$$SV \quad = \quad 50 \text{ mL}$$
$$BSA \quad = \quad 1.1 \text{ m}^2$$

Calculate the left ventricular stroke work (*LVSW*) and its index (*LVSWI*).

$$
\begin{aligned}
LVSW &= (BP_{\text{systolic}} - PCWP) \times SV \times 0.0136 \\
&= (100 - 20) \times 50 \times 0.0136 \\
&= 80 \times 50 \times 0.0136 \\
&= 4000 \times 0.0136 \\
&= 54.4 \text{ g} \cdot \text{m/beat}
\end{aligned}
$$

$$
\begin{aligned}
LVSWI &= \frac{LVSW}{BSA} \\
&= \frac{54.4}{1.1} \\
&= 49.45 \text{ g} \cdot \text{m/beat/m}^2
\end{aligned}
$$

**EXERCISE**

Given: $BP$  = 140/70 mm Hg

$PCWP$ = 20 mm Hg

$SV$  = 45 mL

$BSA$  = 1.5 m$^2$

Calculate the *LVSW* and *LVSWI*.

[Answer: *LVSW* = 73.44 g · m/beat; *LVSWI* = 48.96 g · m/beat/m$^2$]

**REFERENCES**   Bustin; Des Jardins

**SEE**   *Stroke Work: Right Ventricular (RVSW) and Index (RVSWI); Appendix G: Hemodynamic Normal Ranges.*

## Self-Assessment Questions

**72a.** Calculation of the left ventricular stroke work (*LVSW*) and left ventricular stroke work index (*LVSWI*) does not require measurement of

(A) systolic blood pressure

(B) diastolic blood pressure

(C) pulmonary capillary wedge pressure

(D) stroke volume

(E) body surface area

**72b.** The equation for calculating the left ventricular stroke work (*LVSW*) is

(A) $(BP_{systolic} + PCWP) \times SV$

(B) $(BP_{diastolic} + PCWP) \times SV \times 0.0136$

(C) $\dfrac{BP_{systolic} - PCWP}{SV \times 0.0136}$

(D) $(BP_{systolic} - PCWP) \times SV \times 0.0136$

(E) $(BP_{systolic} - PCWP) \times SV$

**72c.** Given: $BP_{systolic}$ = 112 mm Hg, $PCWP$ = 10 mm Hg, $SV$ = 60 mL. What is the calculated left ventricular stroke work (*LVSW*)?

(A) 77.4 g · m/beat

(B) 80.1 g · m/beat

(C) 83.2 g · m/beat

(D) 89.7 g · m/beat

(E) 91.8 g · m/beat

72d. A patient whose estimated body surface area is 1.4 m$^2$ has the following hemodynamic values: $BP_{\text{systolic}}$ = 103 mm Hg, $PCWP$ = 15 mm Hg, $SV$ = 50 mL. What is the patient's left ventricular stroke work index (*LVSWI*)?

(A) 42.7 g · m/beat/m$^2$

(B) 45.5 g · m/beat/m$^2$

(C) 50.6 g · m/beat/m$^2$

(D) 59.8 g · m/beat/m$^2$

(E) 70.1 g · m/beat/m$^2$

72e. The hemodynamic values for a patient (body surface area = 1.3 m$^2$) in the coronary care unit are as follows: $BP$ = 133/65 mm Hg, $CVP$ = 4 mm Hg, $PAP$ = 28 mm Hg, $PCWP$ = 15 mm Hg, $SV$ = 55 mL. What is the patient's left ventricular stroke work (*LVSW*) and index (*LVSWI*)?

(A) $LVSW$ = 79.5 g · m/beat; $LVSWI$ = 61.1 g · m/beat/m$^2$

(B) $LVSW$ = 88.3 g · m/beat; $LVSWI$ = 61.1 g · m/beat/m$^2$

(C) $LVSW$ = 88.3 g · m/beat; $LVSWI$ = 67.9 g · m/beat/m$^2$

(D) $LVSW$ = 93.7 g · m/beat; $LVSWI$ = 67.9 g · m/beat/m$^2$

(E) $LVSW$ = 93.7 g · m/beat; $LVSWI$ = 72.1 g · m/beat/m$^2$

# CHAPTER

# 73
# Stroke Work:
# Right Ventricular (*RVSW*)
# and Index (*RVSWI*)

## NOTES

Right ventricular stroke work (*RVSW*) reflects the work of the right heart in providing perfusion through the pulmonary circulation. *RVSW* is directly related to the pulmonary vascular resistance, myocardial mass, and the volume and viscosity of the blood. In addition, tachycardia, hypoxemia, and poor contractility of the heart may further increase the stroke work of the right heart.

The constant 0.0136 in the equation is used to convert mm Hg/mL to gram · meters (g · m).

The right ventricular stroke work index (*RVSWI*) is used to equalize the stroke work to a person's body size. In the example shown, an apparently normal *RVSW* may be low for a large person after indexing (normal *RVSW*, low *RVSWI*).

## EQUATION 1

$$RVSW = (PA_{systolic} - \overline{RA}) \times SV \times 0.0136$$

## EQUATION 2

$$RVSWI = \frac{RVSW}{BSA}$$

$RVSW$ : Right ventricular stroke work in g · m/beat
$RVSWI$ : Right ventricular stroke work index in g · m/beat/m$^2$
$PA_{systolic}$ : Systolic pulmonary artery pressure in mm Hg
$\overline{RA}$ : Mean right atrial pressure in mm Hg
$SV$ : Stroke volume in mL
$BSA$ : Body surface area in m$^2$

## NORMAL VALUES

$RVSW$ = 10 to 15 g · m/beat
$RVSWI$ = 7 to 12 g · m/beat/m$^2$

## EXAMPLE

Given: $PA_{systolic}$ = 18 mm Hg
$\overline{RA}$ = 4 mm Hg
$SV$ = 60 mL
$BSA$ = 1.9 m$^2$

Calculate the right ventricular stroke work (*RVSW*) and its index (*RVSWI*)

$$RVSW = (PA_{systolic} - \overline{RA}) \times SV \times 0.0136$$
$$= (18 - 4) \times 60 \times 0.0136$$
$$= 14 \times 60 \times 0.0136$$
$$= 840 \times 0.0136$$
$$= 11.42 \text{ g} \cdot \text{m/beat}$$

$$RVSWI = \frac{RVSW}{BSA}$$
$$= \frac{11.42}{1.9}$$
$$= 6.01 \text{ g} \cdot \text{m} / \text{beat} / \text{m}^2$$

**EXERCISE**

Given: $PA_{\text{systolic}}$ = 20 mm Hg
$\overline{RA}$ = 6 mm Hg
$SV$ = 56 mL
$BSA$ = 1.2 m$^2$

Calculate the *RVSW* and *RVSWI*.

[Answer: $RVSW = 10.66$ g · m/beat; $RVSWI = 8.88$ g · m/beat/m$^2$]

**REFERENCE**

Bustin

**SEE**

*Stroke Work: Left Ventricular (LVSW) and Index (LVSWI); Appendix G: Hemodynamic Normal Ranges.*

## Self-Assessment Questions

73a. Which of the following measurements is not required for calculating the right ventricular stroke work (*RVSW*) and right ventricular stroke work index (*RVSWI*)?

(A) mean right atrial pressure

(B) systolic pulmonary artery pressure

(C) stroke volume

(D) systemic artery pressure

(E) body surface area

73b. The equation for calculating the right ventricular stroke work (*RVSW*) is

(A) $(PA_{\text{diastolic}} - \overline{RA}) \times SV$

(B) $(PA_{\text{diastolic}} + \overline{RA}) \times SV \times 0.0136$

(C) $(PA_{\text{systolic}} + \overline{RA}) \times SV$

(D) $(PA_{\text{systolic}} - \overline{RA}) \times SV \times 0.0136$

(E) $\dfrac{PA_{\text{systolic}} - \overline{RA}}{SV \times 0.0136}$

73c. Given: $PA_{\text{systolic}} = 20$ mm Hg, $\overline{RA} = 3$ mm Hg, $SV = 55$ mL. What is the calculated right ventricular stroke work (*RVSW*)?

(A) 11.4 g · m/beat

(B) 12.7 g · m/beat

(C) 13.9 g · m/beat

(D) 15.2 g · m/beat

(E) 16.5 g · m/beat

73d. Given: $PA_{systolic} = 22$ mm Hg, $\overline{RA} = 6$ mm Hg, $SV = 45$ mL, $BSA = 1.1$ m$^2$. Calculate the right ventricular stroke work index (*RVSWI*).

(A) $8.9$ g · m/beat/m$^2$

(B) $9.1$ g · m/beat/m$^2$

(D) $9.3$ g · m/beat/m$^2$

(D) $9.5$ g · m/beat/m$^2$

(E) $9.7$ g · m/beat/m$^2$

73e. A patient whose estimated body surface area is $1.2$ m$^2$ has the following hemodynamic values: $PA_{systolic} = 18$ mm Hg, $\overline{RA} = 3$ mm Hg, $SV = 60$ mL. What is the patient's right ventricular stroke work (*RVSW*) and right ventricular stroke work index (*RVSWI*)?

(A) $RVSW = 9.8$ g · m/beat; $RVSWI = 8.2$ g · m/beat/m$^2$

(B) $RVSW = 10.3$ g · m/beat; $RVSWI = 8.6$ g · m/beat/m$^2$

(C) $RVSW = 11.6$ g · m/beat; $RVSWI = 9.7$ g · m/beat/m$^2$

(D) $RVSW = 12.2$ g · m/beat; $RVSWI = 10.2$ g · m/beat/m$^2$

(E) $RVSW = 13.5$ g · m/beat; $RVSWI = 11.3$ g · m/beat/m$^2$

73f. A patient in the intensive care unit whose body surface area is about $1.4$ m$^2$ has the following hemodynamic values: $PAP = 33/18$ mm Hg; $\overline{RA} = 6$ mm Hg, $SV = 65$ mL. What is the patient's right ventricular stroke work (*RVSW*) and index (*RVSWI*)? Is the index normal?

(A) $RVSW = 23.9$ g · m/beat; $RVSWI = 16.4$ g · m/beat/m$^2$; normal

(B) $RVSW = 23.9$ g · m/beat; $RVSWI = 17.1$ g · m/beat/m$^2$; abnormal

(C) $RVSW = 24.5$ g · m/beat; $RVSWI = 17.5$ g · m/beat/m$^2$; normal

(D) $RVSW = 24.5$ g · m/beat; $RVSWI = 17.1$ g · m/beat/m$^2$; abnormal

(E) $RVSW = 25.3$ g · m/beat; $RVSWI = 18.1$ g · m/beat/m$^2$; abnormal

CHAPTER

# 74
# Temperature Conversion
# (°C to °F)

## NOTES

Temperature conversion calculations are often done in pulmonary function and blood gas laboratories where a conversion chart is not readily available. It is essential to memorize the equation. In the Example, conversion of normal body temperature (from 37 °C to 98.6 °F) was done. If you are unsure of the °C to °F temperature conversion equation, you may first use these two numbers to check for its accuracy.

The temperature constant $\frac{9}{5}$ can be substituted by 1.8 in Celsius to Fahrenheit conversions.

## EQUATION

$$°F = \left(°C \times \frac{9}{5}\right) + 32$$

°F  :  degrees Fahrenheit
°C  :  degrees Celsius

## EXAMPLE

Given: °C = 37
Calculate the degrees Fahrenheit.

$$°F = \left(°C \times \frac{9}{5}\right) + 32$$

$$= \left(37 \times \frac{9}{5}\right) + 32$$

$$= \left(\frac{333}{5}\right) + 32$$

$$= 66.6 + 32$$

$$= 98.6$$

## EXERCISE 1

Given: °C = 25
Find the degrees Fahrenheit.

[Answer: °F = 77]

## EXERCISE 2

Given: °C = 39
Find the degrees Fahrenheit.

[Answer: °F = 102.2]

## REFERENCE

Scanlan

## SEE

*Temperature Conversion (°F to °C).*

## Self-Assessment Questions

74a.  Given: °C = 25. Calculate the degrees Fahrenheit.

(A) 70 °F

(B) 73 °F

(C) 77 °F

(D) 79 °F

(E) 81 °F

74b.  What is the normal body temperature (37 °C) in degrees Fahrenheit?

(A) 96.2 °F

(B) 97.3 °F

(C) 98.1 °F

(D) 98.6 °F

(E) 99.4 °F

74c.  The skin temperature of a neonate is recorded as 36 °C. What is its equivalent in degrees Fahrenheit?

(A) 96.8 °F

(B) 97.4 °F

(C) 98.3 °F

(D) 98.9 °F

(E) 99.5 °F

74d.  The freezing point of water is 0 °C. In degrees Fahrenheit, it is the same as

(A) 0 °F

(B) 0.56 °F

(C) 1.8 °F

(D) 21 °F

(E) 32 °F

CHAPTER

# 75
# Temperature Conversion (°C to K)

## NOTES

In respiratory care, the Kelvin (K or °T) temperature scale is primarily used in gas law calculations (i.e., Boyle's law, Charles' law, Gay-Lussac's law, and Combined Gas Law).

Kelvin temperature is also called the absolute temperature because molecular activity of gases theoretically stops at 0 K (– 273 °C). In the Equation, it is essential to remember the constant number 273.

For temperature conversion from Fahrenheit (°F) to kelvins (K), change °F to °C and then use the Equation to solve for K.

## EQUATION

$K = °C + 273$

K : kelvins
°C : degrees Celsius

## EXAMPLE

Given: °C = 37
Calculate the Kelvin equivalent.

$$K = °C + 273$$
$$= 37 + 273$$
$$= 310$$

## EXERCISE 1

Given: °C = 25
Find the Kelvin equivalent.

[Answer: K = 298]

## EXERCISE 2

Given: °C = 39
Find the Kelvin equivalent.

[Answer: K = 312]

## REFERENCE

Scanlan

# Self-Assessment Questions

75a.  The equation to convert a known temperature to kelvins is

(A) 273 – °C

(B) °C + 273

(C) 273 – °F

(D) °F + 273

(E) °F – 273

75b.  Given: °C = 25. Calculate the kelvin equivalent.

(A) 360

(B) 325

(C) 312

(D) 304

(E) 298

75c.  Given: °F = 88 (31 °C). Calculate the kelvin equivalent.

(A) 360

(B) 325

(C) 312

(D) 304

(E) 298

75d.  A gas volume is measured at 26 °C. Find its equivalent in kelvins (K) for temperature correction with the Combined Gas Law.

(A) 247 K

(B) 288 K

(C) 299 K

(D) 330 K

(E) 352 K

75e.  Which of the following gas temperatures is the same as 310 K?

(A) 35 °C

(B) 37 °C

(C) 39 °C

(D) 94 °F

(E) 95 °F

# 76
# Temperature Conversion (°F to °C)

## NOTES

Temperature conversion calculations are often done in pulmonary function and blood gas laboratories where a conversion chart is not readily available. It is essential to memorize the equation. In the Example, conversion of normal body temperature (from 98.6 °F to 37 °C) was done. If you are unsure of the °F to °C temperature conversion equation, you may first use these two numbers to check for its accuracy.

To convert Fahrenheit to kelvins, first change Fahrenheit to Celsius and then change to kelvins.

## EQUATION

$$°C = (°F - 32) \times \frac{5}{9}$$

°C : degrees Celsius
°F : degrees Fahrenheit

## EXAMPLE

Given: °F = 98.6
Calculate the degrees Celsius.

$$°C = (°F - 32) \times \frac{5}{9}$$

$$= (98.6 - 32) \times \frac{5}{9}$$

$$= (66.6) \times \frac{5}{9}$$

$$= \frac{333}{9}$$

$$= 37$$

## EXERCISE

Given: °F = 100
Find the degrees Celsius.

[Answer: °C = 37.77 or 37.8]

## REFERENCE

Scanlan

## SEE

*Temperature Conversion (°C to K); Temperature Conversion (°C to °F).*

## *Self-Assessment Questions*

76a.  A patient has an oral temperature of 99.2 °F. It is the same as

(A) 36.8 °C

(B) 37.3 °C

(C) 37.7 °C

(D) 38.1 °C

(E) 38.9 °C

76b.  The rectal temperature of a neonate is 101.5 °F. It is equal to

(A) 37.4 °C

(B) 37.7 °C

(C) 38.6 °C

(D) 39.0 °C

(E) 39.5 °C

76c.  A room temperature of 78 °F is the same as

(A) 23.3 °C

(B) 23.7 °C

(C) 24.4 °C

(D) 25.6 °C

(E) 26.9 °C

# 77

# Tidal Volume Based on Flow and *I* Time

*NOTES*

The tidal volume delivered by a pressure-limited ventilator is directly related to the flow rate and inspiratory time (*I* time), providing the peak inspiratory pressure is sufficient. A higher flow rate or longer *I* time usually yields a larger tidal volume in the absence of severe airway obstruction or lung parenchymal disease.

However, a prolonged *I* time increases the mean airway pressure and the likelihood of barotrauma. Therefore, as more ventilation is needed when using a pressure-limited ventilator, one should evaluate and consider other options such as increasing the peak inspiratory pressure, ventilator frequency, or flow rate. While these options carry similar complications, a combination of these options may help to improve ventilation with minimal side effects.

## EQUATION

$V_T = \text{Flow} \times I \text{ time}$

$V_T$ : Tidal volume in mL
Flow : Flow rate in mL/sec
*I* time : Inspiratory time in sec

## EXAMPLE

Given: Flow         = 8 L/min
      Inspiratory time = 0.5 sec
Calculate the approximate tidal volume.
First change the flow rate from L/min to mL/sec. Flow rate at 8 L/min is the same as 8000 mL/60 sec or 133 mL/sec.

$$V_T = \text{Flow} \times I \text{ time}$$
$$= 133 \text{ mL/sec} \times 0.5 \text{ sec}$$
$$= 66.5 \text{ mL}$$

## EXERCISE

Given the following settings on a pressure-limited ventilator: Flow = 6 L/min; inspiratory time = 0.4 sec. What is the approximate tidal volume based on these settings?

[Answer: $V_T = 40$ mL]

## REFERENCE

Whitaker

## SEE

*Mean Airway Pressure (MAWP).*

## Self-Assessment Questions

77a. Given: flow = 7 L/min, inspiratory time = 0.5 sec. Calculate the delivered tidal volume based on these settings on a pressure-limited ventilator.

   (A) 45 mL

   (B) 47 mL

   (C) 50 mL

   (D) 53 mL

   (E) 58 mL

77b. The following settings are used on a pressure-limited ventilator: flow = 8 L/min, inspiratory time = 0.4 sec. Calculate the delivered tidal volume on these settings.

   (A) 45 mL

   (B) 47 mL

   (C) 50 mL

   (D) 53 mL

   (E) 58 mL

77c. Given the following flow rate (Flow) and inspiratory time (*I* time). Which set of values provides the lowest delivered tidal volume?

| | Flow (L/min) | *I* time (sec) |
|---|---|---|
| (A) | 7 | 0.3 |
| (B) | 7 | 0.4 |
| (C) | 6 | 0.4 |
| (D) | 6 | 0.5 |
| (E) | 7 | 0.5 |

77d. The following sets of data are found on the flow sheet of an infant ventilator over a 3-day period. Which set of values has the highest calculated tidal volume?

| | Flow (L/min) | *I* time (sec) |
|---|---|---|
| (A) | 6 | 0.4 |
| (B) | 7 | 0.4 |
| (C) | 8 | 0.4 |
| (D) | 6 | 0.5 |
| (E) | 7 | 0.5 |

77e. The physician asks you to make changes on an infant ventilator so as to increase the tidal volume. You would

   (A) decrease the PEEP

   (B) decrease the $F_IO_2$

   (C) increase the expiratory time

   (D) increase the *CPAP*

   (E) increase the inspiratory time

# 78
# Time Constant

## NOTES

Time constant (*t*) is defined as the time needed to inflate a lung region to 60% of its filling capacity. It is directly related to the resistance (elastic lung parenchymal resistance and non-elastic airway resistance) and the compliance (lung and chest-wall compliance). When resistance and compliance are treated separately, an increase of time constant reflects an increase in resistance, or compliance, or both. In other words, the lungs of a patient with high resistance or compliance take a longer time to inflate. Likewise, when the resistance and compliance are low, the time needed to inflate the lungs is shorter.

However, the relationship between resistance and compliance may mask the changes of time constant. For example, atelectasis causes a *decrease* in lung compliance but an *increase* in elastic lung parenchymal resistance. For this reason, opposing changes of compliance and resistance may result in an unchanged time constant.

A better way to evaluate the changes in resistance and compliance is to compare the dynamic and static compliance values.

## EQUATION

$t = R \times C$

$t$ : Time constant in seconds

$R$ : Resistance in cm $H_2O$ / L / sec

$C$ : Compliance in L / cm $H_2O$

## NORMAL VALUE

Use serial measurements to establish trend.

## EXAMPLE

A patient who is on mechanical ventilation has a total resistance of 5 cm $H_2O$ / L / sec and a compliance of 0.08 L / cm $H_2O$. What is the calculated time constant?

$$t = R \times C$$
$$= 5 \times 0.08$$
$$= 0.4 \sec$$

## EXERCISE

A patient who is being mechanically ventilated has a resistance of 6 cm $H_2O$ / L / sec and a compliance of 0.06 L / cm $H_2O$. What is the calculated time constant?

[Answer: $t = 0.36$ sec]

## REFERENCES

Des Jardins; Dupuis; Rattenborg

## SEE

*Compliance: Dynamic ($C_{dyn}$); Compliance: Static ($C_{st}$).*

# Self-Assessment Questions

78a. A patient who is on mechanical ventilation has a total resistance of 8 cm $H_2O/L/sec$ and a compliance of 0.06 L/cm $H_2O$. What is the calculated time constant?

(A) 0.20 sec

(B) 0.48 sec

(C) 0.75 sec

(D) 1.33 sec

(E) 2.00 sec

78b. A patient who is being mechanically ventilated has a total resistance of 7 cm $H_2O/L/sec$ and a compliance of 0.033 L/cm $H_2O$. What is the calculated time constant?

(A) 0.15 sec

(B) 0.19 sec

(C) 0.23 sec

(D) 0.27 sec

(E) 0.29 sec

78c. The pulmonary dynamics of a ventilator-dependent patient in the surgical intensive care unit are as follows: resistance = 12 cm $H_2O/L/sec$, compliance = 0.02 L/cm $H_2O$. What is the time constant based on the values provided?

(A) 0.06 sec

(B) 0.02 sec

(C) 0.2 sec

(D) 0.24 sec

(E) 0.6 sec

CHAPTER

# 79
# Vascular Resistance: Pulmonary

*NOTES*

Pulmonary vascular resistance (*PVR*) reflects the resistance of pulmonary vessel to blood flow. A Swan-Ganz catheter is required to obtain the $\overline{PA}$ and *PCWP* readings. The cardiac output must also be known to calculate the *PVR*.

The constant value 80 in the equation is used to convert the *PVR* to absolute resistance units, dynes $\cdot$ sec/cm$^5$.

Under normal conditions, the *PVR* is about one-sixth of the systemic vascular resistance. An abnormally high *PVR* may indicate pulmonary vascular problems such as pulmonary hypertension, reduction of capillary bed, and pulmonary embolism. An extremely low *PVR* may be associated with reduction in circulating blood volume such as hypovolemic shock.

See Tables 11 and 12 for factors that change the pulmonary vascular resistance.

## EQUATION

$$PVR = (\overline{PA} - PCWP) \times \frac{80}{CO}$$

$PVR$ : Pulmonary vascular resistance in dyne $\cdot$ sec/cm$^5$
$\overline{PA}$ : Mean pulmonary artery pressure in mm Hg
$PCWP$ : Pulmonary capillary wedge pressure in mm Hg
$CO$ : Cardiac output in L/min ($\dot{Q}_T$)

### TABLE 11. Factors That Increase Pulmonary Vascular Resistance (*PVR*)

**Chemical Stimuli**
Decreased alveolar oxygenation
(alveolar hypoxia)
Decreased pH (acidemia)
Increased $PCO_2$ (hypercapnia)

**Pharmacologic Agents**
Epinephrine (Adrenalin®)
Norepinephrine (Levophed®, Levarterenol®)
Dobutamine (Dobutrex®)
Dopamine (Intropin®)
Phenylephrine (Neo-Synephrine®)

**Hyperinflation of Lungs**
Mechanical ventilation
Continuous Positive Airway Pressure (CPAP)
Positive End-Expiratory Pressure (PEEP)

**Pathologic Factors**
Vascular blockage
Pulmonary emboli
Air bubble
Tumor mass

Vascular wall disease
Sclerosis
Endateritis
Polyarteritis
Scleroderma

Vascular destruction
Emphysema
Pulmonary interstitial fibrosis

Vascular compression
Pneumothorax
Hemothorax
Tumor mass

**Humoral Substances**
Histamine
Angiotensin
Fibrinopeptides
Prostaglandin $F_{2\alpha}$
Serotonin

From Des Jardins, T.R., *Cardiopulmonary Anatomy and Physiology: Essentials for Respiratory Care*, 3rd ed. Albany, NY: Delmar Publishers, 1998.

**TABLE 12.    Factors That Decrease Pulmonary Vascular Resistance (*PVR*)**

| PHARMACOLOGIC AGENTS | HUMORAL SUBSTANCES |
|---|---|
| Oxygen | Acetylcholine |
| Isoproterenol (Isuprel®) | Bradykinin |
| Aminophylline | Prostaglandin E |
| Calcium-blocking agent | Prostacyclin (prostaglandin $I_2$) |

From Des Jardins, T.R., *Cardiopulmonary Anatomy and Physiology: Essentials for Respiratory Care,* 3rd ed. Albany, NY: Delmar Publishers, 1998.

## NORMAL VALUE

$PVR = 50$ to $150$ dyne $\cdot$ sec $/ \text{cm}^5$

## EXAMPLE

A patient has the following measurements. What is the calculated pulmonary vascular resistance (*PVR*)?

$\overline{PA}$ = 22 mm Hg

$PCWP$ = 6 mm Hg

$CO$ = 4.0 L / min

$$PVR = (\overline{PA} - PCWP) \times \frac{80}{CO}$$

$$= (22 - 6) \times \frac{80}{4.0}$$

$$= 16 \times \frac{80}{4.0}$$

$$= \frac{1280}{4}$$

$$= 320 \text{ dyne} \cdot \text{sec} / \text{cm}^5$$

## EXERCISE

What is the patient's pulmonary vascular resistance (*PVR*) if the following measurements are recorded?

$\overline{PA}$ = 24 mm Hg

$PCWP$ = 7 mm Hg

$CO$ = 5.0 L / min

[Answer: $PVR = 272$ dyne $\cdot$ sec $/ \text{cm}^5$]

## REFERENCES

Bustin; Des Jardins

## SEE

*Appendix G: Hemodynamic Normal Ranges.*

## Self-Assessment Questions

79a. In order to calculate the pulmonary vascular resistance, all of the following procedures or parameters are necessary with the *exception* of

(A) Swan-Ganz catheter

(B) mean pulmonary artery pressure

(C) pulmonary capillary wedge pressure

(D) cardiac output

(E) systemic artery pressure

79b. A patient has the following measurements: mean pulmonary artery pressure = 20 mm Hg, pulmonary capillary wedge pressure = 7 mm Hg, cardiac output = 5.0 L/min. What is the pulmonary vascular resistance (*PVR*)?

(A) 180 dynes $\cdot$ sec/cm$^5$

(B) 195 dynes $\cdot$ sec/cm$^5$

(C) 208 dynes $\cdot$ sec/cm$^5$

(D) 223 dynes $\cdot$ sec/cm$^5$

(E) 268 dynes $\cdot$ sec/cm$^5$

79c. The following hemodynamic measurements are obtained from a patient in the intensive care unit. What is the calculated pulmonary vascular resistance (*PVR*)?

Mean pulmonary artery pressure =   18 mm Hg

Pulmonary capillary wedge pressure =   8 mm Hg

Cardiac output   =   4.5 L/min

(A) 146 dynes $\cdot$ sec/cm$^5$

(B) 155 dynes $\cdot$ sec/cm$^5$

(C) 160 dynes $\cdot$ sec/cm$^5$

(D) 178 dynes $\cdot$ sec/cm$^5$

(E) 183 dynes $\cdot$ sec/cm$^5$

79d. Calculate the patient's pulmonary vascular resistance (*PVR*) with the following measurements obtained during a hemodynamic study.

Mean pulmonary artery pressure =   20 mm Hg

Pulmonary capillary wedge pressure =   6 mm Hg

Cardiac output   =   5.1 L/min

(A) 210 dynes $\cdot$ sec/cm$^5$

(B) 220 dynes $\cdot$ sec/cm$^5$

(C) 230 dynes $\cdot$ sec/cm$^5$

(D) 240 dynes $\cdot$ sec/cm$^5$

(E) 250 dynes $\cdot$ sec/cm$^5$

# CHAPTER

# *80*

# Vascular Resistance: Systemic

## NOTES

Systemic vascular resistance (*SVR*) reflects the resistance of systemic vessel to blood flow. The *MAP* (mean arterial pressure) in the equation is a measured value, or it may be estimated by using the systolic and diastolic pressure readings.* The right atrial pressure and the cardiac output must also be known to calculate the *SVR*. The constant value 80 in the equation is used to convert the *SVR* to absolute resistance units dyne · sec/cm$^5$.

The normal *SVR* is about six times the pulmonary vascular resistance. An abnormally high *SVR* may indicate systemic vasoconstriction (e.g., response to hypovolemia). An abnormally low *SVR* may be indicative of peripheral vasodilation (e.g., early stages of septic shock).

See Table 13 for factors that change the systemic vascular resistance.

## EQUATION

$$SVR = (MAP - \overline{RA}) \times \frac{80}{CO}$$

$SVR$ : Systemic vascular resistance in dyne · sec/cm$^5$
$MAP$ : Mean arterial pressure in mm Hg*
$\overline{RA}$ : Mean right atrial pressure in mm Hg
$CO$ : Cardiac output in L/min ($\dot{Q}_T$)

## NORMAL VALUE

$$SVR = 800 \text{ to } 1500 \text{ dyne} \cdot \text{sec/cm}^5$$

## EXAMPLE

A patient has the following measurements. What is the calculated systemic vascular resistance (*SVR*)?

$MAP = 70$ mm Hg
$\overline{RA} = 8$ mm Hg
$CO = 5.0$ L/min

$$SVR = (MAP - \overline{RA}) \times \frac{80}{CO}$$

$$= (70 - 8) \times \frac{80}{5.0}$$

$$= 62 \times \frac{80}{5.0}$$

$$= \frac{4960}{5}$$

$$= 992 \text{ dyne} \cdot \text{sec/cm}^5$$

## EXERCISE

What is the patient's systemic vascular resistance (*SVR*) if the following measurements are recorded?

$MAP = 76$ mm Hg
$\overline{RA} = 6$ mm Hg
$CO = 5.0$ L/min

[Answer: $SVR = 1120$ dyne · sec/cm$^5$]

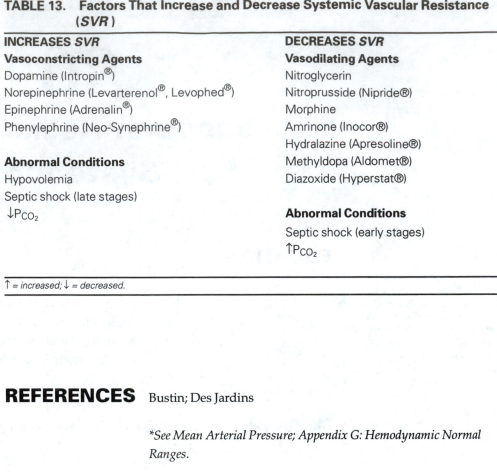

**TABLE 13. Factors That Increase and Decrease Systemic Vascular Resistance (SVR)**

| INCREASES SVR | DECREASES SVR |
|---|---|
| **Vasoconstricting Agents** | **Vasodilating Agents** |
| Dopamine (Intropin®) | Nitroglycerin |
| Norepinephrine (Levarterenol®, Levophed®) | Nitroprusside (Nipride®) |
| Epinephrine (Adrenalin®) | Morphine |
| Phenylephrine (Neo-Synephrine®) | Amrinone (Inocor®) |
| | Hydralazine (Apresoline®) |
| **Abnormal Conditions** | Methyldopa (Aldomet®) |
| Hypovolemia | Diazoxide (Hyperstat®) |
| Septic shock (late stages) | |
| $\downarrow P_{CO_2}$ | **Abnormal Conditions** |
| | Septic shock (early stages) |
| | $\uparrow P_{CO_2}$ |

$\uparrow$ = increased; $\downarrow$ = decreased.

**REFERENCES**  Bustin; Des Jardins

*See Mean Arterial Pressure; Appendix G: Hemodynamic Normal Ranges.*

# Self-Assessment Questions

80a. To calculate a patient's systemic vascular resistance (*SVR*), all of the following procedures or parameters are needed *except*

    (A) pulmonary artery pressure

    (B) arterial catheter

    (C) mean arterial pressure

    (D) mean right atrial pressure

    (E) cardiac output

80b. A patient has the following measurements: mean arterial pressure = 70 mm Hg, mean right atrial pressure = 10 mm Hg, cardiac output = 4.0 L/min. What is the systemic vascular resistance (*SVR*)?

    (A) 900 dynes · sec/cm$^5$

    (B) 1000 dynes · sec/cm$^5$

    (C) 1100 dynes · sec/cm$^5$

    (D) 1200 dynes · sec/cm$^5$

    (E) 1300 dynes · sec/cm$^5$

80c. The following hemodynamic information is obtained from a patient's chart. What is the calculated systemic vascular resistance ($SVR$)?

Mean arterial pressure = 62 mm Hg
Mean right atrial pressure = 6 mm Hg
Cardiac output = 4.2 L/min

(A) 107 dynes · sec/cm$^5$

(B) 667 dynes · sec/cm$^5$

(C) 1067 dynes · sec/cm$^5$

(D) 1120 dynes · sec/cm$^5$

(E) 1226 dynes · sec/cm$^5$

80d. What is the patient's systemic vascular resistance ($SVR$) if the following measurements are recorded? $MAP = 55$ mm Hg, $\overline{RA} = 5$ mm Hg, $CO = 3.8$ L/min.

(A) 105 dynes · sec/cm$^5$

(B) 226 dynes · sec/cm$^5$

(C) 904 dynes · sec/cm$^5$

(D) 998 dynes · sec/cm$^5$

(E) 1053 dynes · sec/cm$^5$

80e. The following hemodynamic measurements are obtained from a patient in the intensive care unit. What are the calculated pulmonary vascular resistance ($PVR$) and systemic vascular resistance ($SVR$)?

Mean pulmonary arterial pressure = 20 mm Hg
Pulmonary capillary wedge pressure = 7 mm Hg
Mean arterial pressure = 70 mm Hg
Mean right atrial pressure = 4 mm Hg
Cardiac output = 4.2 L/min

(A) $PVR = 226$ dynes · sec/cm$^5$; $SVR = 1257$ dynes · sec/cm$^5$

(B) $PVR = 226$ dynes · sec/cm$^5$; $SVR = 1303$ dynes · sec/cm$^5$

(C) $PVR = 248$ dynes · sec/cm$^5$; $SVR = 1257$ dynes · sec/cm$^5$

(D) $PVR = 248$ dynes · sec/cm$^5$; $SVR = 1303$ dynes · sec/cm$^5$

(E) $PVR = 261$ dynes · sec/cm$^5$; $SVR = 1442$ dynes · sec/cm$^5$

# CHAPTER

# 81
# Ventilator Rate Needed for a Desired $P_aCO_2$

**EQUATION 1**

$$\text{New rate} = \frac{\text{Rate} \times P_aCO_2}{\text{Desired } P_aCO_2*}$$

**EQUATION 2**

$$\text{New rate} = \frac{(\text{Rate} \times P_aCO_2) \times (V_T - V_D)}{\text{Desired } P_aCO_2 \times (\text{New } V_T - \text{New } V_D)**}$$

| | | |
|---|---|---|
| New rate | : | Ventilator rate needed for a desired $P_aCO_2$ |
| Rate | : | Original ventilator rate / min |
| $P_aCO_2$ | : | Original arterial carbon dioxide tension in mm Hg |
| Desired $P_aCO_2$ | : | Desired arterial carbon dioxide tension in mm Hg |
| $V_T$ | : | Original tidal volume |
| $V_D$ | : | Original deadspace volume |
| New $V_T$ | : | New tidal volume |
| New $V_D$ | : | New deadspace volume |

**NORMAL VALUE**

Set rate to provide eucapnic (patient's normal) ventilation.

**EXAMPLE 1**

When tidal volume and deadspace volume remain unchanged.

The $P_aCO_2$ of a patient is 55 mm Hg at a ventilator rate of 10 / min. What should be the ventilator rate if a $P_aCO_2$ of 40 mm Hg is desired assuming the ventilator tidal volume and spontaneous ventilation are stable?

$$\text{New rate} = \frac{(\text{Rate} \times P_aCO_2)}{\text{Desired } P_aCO_2}$$

$$= \frac{(10 \times 55)}{40}$$

$$= \frac{550}{40}$$

$$= 13.75 \text{ or } 14/\text{min}$$

*When tidal volume and deadspace volume stay unchanged.*

**When tidal volume or deadspace volume is changed.*

*NOTES (cont.)*

If the ventilator tidal volume remains unchanged, new $V_T$ = $V_T$. If the mechanical deadspace remains unchanged, new $V_D$ = $V_D$.

## EXAMPLE 2

When tidal volume or deadspace volume is changed.

A patient has a $P_a CO_2$ of 25 mm Hg at a ventilator tidal volume of 800 mL, 0 mL added circuit deadspace, and a rate of 10/min. If the ventilator tidal volume is changed to 780 mL and if 50 mL of mechanical deadspace is added to the ventilator circuit, what should be the new ventilator rate for a desired $P_a CO_2$ of 40 mm Hg?

$$\text{New rate} = \frac{(\text{Rate} \times P_a CO_2) \times (V_T - V_D)}{\text{Desired } P_a CO_2 \times (\text{New } V_T - \text{New } V_D)}$$

$$= \frac{(10 \times 25) \times (800 - 0)}{40 \times (780 - 50)}$$

$$= \frac{(250) \times (800)}{40 \times (730)}$$

$$= \frac{200,000}{29,200}$$

$$= 6.85 \text{ or } 7/\text{min}$$

## EXERCISE 1

At a ventilator rate of 8/min, a patient's $P_a CO_2$ is 55 mm Hg. Calculate the new ventilator rate if a $P_a CO_2$ of 40 mm Hg is desired (assuming the ventilator tidal volume and spontaneous ventilation remain unchanged).

[Answer: New rate = 11/min]

## EXERCISE 2

A patient has a $P_a CO_2$ of 30 min Hg at a ventilator tidal volume of 700 mL and a rate of 8/min. If 50 mL of mechanical deadspace is added to the ventilator circuit, what should be the new ventilator rate for a desired $P_a CO_2$ of 40 mm Hg? What should be the calculated new rate if no mechanical deadspace is used?

[Answer: New rate = 6.46 or 7/min; new rate without deadspace = 6/min]

## REFERENCES

Barnes; Burton

## Self-Assessment Questions

81a. Given: $P_aCO_2$ = 60 mm Hg, ventilator rate = 12/min. Calculate the estimated ventilator rate for a $P_aCO_2$ of 45 mm Hg (assuming the ventilator tidal volume and spontaneous ventilation are stable).

(A) 14/min

(B) 15/min

(C) 16/min

(D) 17/min

(E) 18/min

81b. Given: $P_aCO_2$ = 30 mm Hg, ventilator rate = 16/min. Calculate the estimated ventilator rate for a $P_aCO_2$ of 40 mm Hg (assuming the ventilator tidal volume and spontaneous ventilation are stable).

(A) 11/min

(B) 12/min

(C) 13/min

(D) 14/min

(E) 15/min

81c. The $P_aCO_2$ of a patient is 48 mm Hg at a ventilator rate of 12/min. What should be the ventilator rate if a $P_aCO_2$ of 36 mm Hg is desired (assuming the ventilator tidal volume and spontaneous ventilation are stable)?

(A) 14/min

(B) 15/min

(C) 16/min

(D) 17/min

(E) 18/min

81d. A patient has a $P_aCO_2$ of 22 mm Hg at a ventilator tidal volume of 850 mL and a rate of 12/min. If 50 mL of mechanical deadspace is added to the ventilator circuit, what should be the new ventilator rate for a desired $P_aCO_2$ of 35 mm Hg?

(A) 7/min

(B) 8/min

(C) 9/min

(D) 10/min

(E) 11/min

81e. A patient has a $P_aCO_2$ of 65 mm Hg at a ventilator tidal volume of 750 mL and a rate of 12/min. If the ventilator tidal volume is changed to 850 mL, what should be the new ventilator rate for a desired $P_aCO_2$ of 40 mm Hg?

(A) 17/min

(B) 16/min

(C) 15/min

(D) 14/min

(E) 13/min

81f. The $P_aCO_2$ of a patient is 28 mm Hg at a ventilator tidal volume of 900 mL and a rate of 16/min. If the ventilator tidal volume is decreased to 800 mL, what should be the new ventilator rate for a desired $P_aCO_2$ of 40 mm Hg?

(A) 17/min

(B) 16/min

(C) 15/min

(D) 14/min

(E) 13/min

# 82

# Weaning Index: Rapid Shallow Breathing (*RSBWI*)

## NOTES

Failure of weaning from mechanical ventilation may be related to a spontaneous breathing pattern that is rapid (high respiratory rate) and shallow (low tidal volume). The ratio of spontaneous respiratory rate and spontaneous tidal volume (in liters) has been used to evaluate the presence and severity of this breathing pattern.

Rapid shallow breathing is quantified as the $f$ (breaths per minute) divided by the $V_T$ in liters. This breathing pattern promotes inefficient, deadspace ventilation. When the $f/V_T$ ratio becomes greater than 100 breaths/min/L, it suggests potential weaning failure. On the other hand, absence of rapid shallow breathing, as defined by an $f/V_T$ ratio of less than 100 breaths/min/L, is a very accurate predictor of weaning success (Yang, 1991).

To measure the $f/V_T$ ratio, the patient is taken off the ventilator and allowed to breathe spontaneously for at least one minute or until a stable breathing pattern has been established. Invalid assumption of the patient's breathing status may occur if measurements are done before the patient reaches a stable spontaneous breathing pattern. In addition, any ventilatory adjuncts such as pressure support ventilation (PSV) and continuous positive airway pressure (CPAP) should not be used in

## EQUATION

$RSBWI = f/V_T$

$RSBWI$:    Rapid Shallow Breathing Weaning Index, in breaths/min/L or cycles/L

$f$    :    Spontaneous respiratory rate in breaths/min (cycles)

$V_T$    :    Spontaneous tidal volume, in liters

## NORMAL VALUE

< 100 breaths/min/L is predictive of weaning success.

## EXAMPLE

A patient who has been on mechanical ventilation is being evaluated for weaning trial. While breathing spontaneously, the minute ventilation is 4.5 L/min at a rate of 18/min.

What is the average spontaneous tidal volume, in liters? What is the calculated Rapid Shallow Breathing Weaning Index ($f/V_T$)? Does this index suggest a successful weaning outcome?

$$\text{Average spontaneous } V_T = \text{minute ventilation / respiratory rate}$$
$$= 4.5 / 18$$
$$= 0.25 \text{ L}$$

$$\text{Rapid Shallow Breathing Weaning Index} = f/V_T$$
$$= 18 / 0.25$$
$$= 72 \text{ breaths/min/L}$$

Since the Rapid Shallow Breathing Weaning Index is less than 100, the calculated index suggests a successful weaning outcome.

## EXERCISE

A mechanically ventilated patient is being evaluated for weaning trial. The spontaneous minute ventilation and spontaneous respiratory rate are 7.6 L/min and 36/min, respectively.

What is the average spontaneous tidal volume, in liters? What is the calculated Rapid Shallow Breathing Weaning Index ($f/V_T$)? Does this index show a successful weaning outcome?

preparing the patient for the *RSBWI* assessment.

The minute expired volume ($V_E$) is measured by a respirometer and the corresponding respiratory frequency ($f$) is recorded. The $V_T$ is calculated by dividing the $V_E$ by $f$. The $f/V_T$ ratio is calculated by dividing the $f$ by $V_T$. Remember, the $V_T$ in the calculations is always expressed in liters.

**ANSWERS**

Average spontaneous $V_T = 0.21$ L
Rapid Shallow Breathing Weaning Index = 171 breaths/min/L
Since the Rapid Shallow Breathing Weaning Index is greater than 100 breaths/min/L, the calculated index suggests a poor weaning outcome.

**REFERENCES**   Tobin, 1986; Yang, 1991.

## Self-Assessment Questions

82a. Successful weaning from mechanical ventilation is likely when the *RSBWI* is:

(A) greater than 100 breaths/min/L

(B) less than 100 breaths/min/L

(C) greater than 100 L

(D) less than 100 L

82b. *RSBWI* requires measurements of the _____ minute ventilation and spontaneous _____.

(A) mechanical, respiratory rate

(B) mechanical, tidal volume

(C) spontaneous, respiratory rate

(D) spontaneous, tidal volume

82c. *RSBWI* is calculated by:

(A) dividing a patient's spontaneous tidal volume by respiratory rate

(B) multiplying a patient's spontaneous tidal volume and respiratory rate

(C) dividing a patient's spontaneous respiratory rate by tidal volume

(D) multiplying a patient's spontaneous minute ventilation and respiratory rate

82d. Given the following measurements: Spontaneous minute ventilation = 4.5 L/min, spontaneous respiratory rate = 23/min. What is the average spontaneous tidal volume, in liters?

(A) 0.196 L

(B) 0.511 L

(C) 1.96 L

(D) 5.11 L

82e. Given the following measurements: Spontaneous minute ventilation = 4.5 L/min, spontaneous respiratory rate = 23/min. What is the calculated *RSBWI*? Does the *RSBWI* indicate a successful outcome?

(A) 110 breaths/min/L. Yes.

(B) 110 breaths/min/L. No.

(C) 117 breaths/min/L. Yes.

(D) 117 breaths/min/L. No.

82f. Given the following measurements: Spontaneous minute ventilation = 4.2

L/min, spontaneous respiratory rate = 17/min. What is the average spontaneous tidal volume, in liters?

(A) 0.247 L

(B) 0.714 L

(C) 2.47 L

(D) 7.14 L

82g. Given the following measurements: Spontaneous minute ventilation = 4.2 L/min, spontaneous respiratory rate = 17/min. What is the calculated *RSBWI*? Does the *RSBWI* indicate a successful outcome?

(A) 24 breaths/min/L. Yes.

(B) 24 breaths/min/L. No.

(C) 69 breaths/min/L. Yes.

(D) 69 breaths/min/L. No.

82h. Mr. Johns, a mechanically ventilated patient, is being evaluated for weaning attempt. His spontaneous minute ventilation and respiratory rate are 5.9 L/min and 22/min, respectively. What is the average spontaneous tidal volume, in liters? What is the calculated Rapid Shallow Breathing Weaning Index ($f / V_T$)? Does the calculated *RSBWI* show a successful weaning outcome?

(A) Average spontaneous $V_T$ = 0.251 L.    *RSBWI* = 87 breaths/min/L. Yes.

(B) Average spontaneous $V_T$ = 0.268 L.    *RSBWI* = 82 breaths/min/L. Yes.

(C) Average spontaneous $V_T$ = 0.251 L.    *RSBWI* =125 breaths/min/L. No.

(D) Average spontaneous $V_T$ = 0.268 L.    *RSBWI* = 125 breaths/min/L. No.

82i. The spontaneous minute ventilation and respiratory rate of a mechanically ventilated patient are 6.2 L/min and 30/min, respectively. Calculate the average spontaneous tidal volume, in liters, and the Rapid Shallow Breathing Weaning Index ($f / V_T$). Does the calculated *RSBWI* indicate a successful weaning outcome?

(A) Average spontaneous $V_T$ = 0.207 L.    *RSBWI* = 90 breaths/min/L. Yes.

(B) Average spontaneous $V_T$ = 0.207 L.    *RSBWI* = 145 breaths/min/L. No.

(C) Average spontaneous $V_T$ = 0.219 L.    *RSBWI* = 90 breaths/min/L. Yes.

(D) Average spontaneous $V_T$ = 0.219 L.    *RSBWI* = 137 breaths/min/L. No.

# *83*
# Weaning Index: Simplified (*SWI*)

## NOTES

The Simplified Weaning Index (*SWI*) is based on the following parameters and measurements obtained during the assist or control mode of mechanical ventilation: Ventilator respiratory rate ($f_{mv}$), peak inspiratory pressure (PIP), PEEP, spontaneous maximum inspiratory pressure (MIP), and $P_aCO_2$ while receiving mechanical ventilation.

When the *SWI* is less than 9/min, it is highly predictive (93%) of weaning success; when the *SWI* is greater than 11/min, there is a 95% probability of weaning failure. *SWI* evaluates a patient's ventilatory endurance and the efficiency of gas exchange. Even though *SWI* is a simplified version of the original weaning index, its simplicity and exclusive use of common parameters make this index a practical method of assessment during routine ventilator care.

## EQUATION

$$SWI = [f_{mv}\,(PIP - PEEP)\,/\,MIP] \times (P_aCO_{2mv}\,/\,40)$$

| | | |
|---|---|---|
| *SWI* | : | Simplified Weaning Index, in units / min |
| $f_{mv}$ | : | Ventilator frequency, in breaths / min. |
| PIP | : | Peak inspiratory pressure, in cm $H_2O$. |
| PEEP | : | Positive end-expiratory pressure, in mm Hg. |
| MIP | : | Maximal inspiratory pressure, in cm $H_2O$. [Ignore negative sign] |
| $P_aCO_{2mv}$ | : | Arterial $CO_2$ tension while on ventilator, in mm Hg. |

## NORMAL VALUE

< 9 / min is predictive of weaning success.
Between 9 / min and 11 / min is predictive of 50% weaning success.
> 11 / min is predictive of weaning failure.

## EXAMPLE

Calculate the simplified weaning index given the following parameters and measurements. Does this index indicate a successful weaning outcome?

$f_{mv}$ = 8 / min, PIP = 50 cm $H_2O$, PEEP = 10 cm $H_2O$, MIP = –30 cm $H_2O$, $P_aCO_{2mv}$ = 45 mm Hg.

$$
\begin{aligned}
SWI &= [f_{mv}\,(PIP - PEEP)\,/\,MIP] \times (P_aCO_{2mv}\,/\,40) \\
&= [8\,(50 - 10)\,/\,30] \times (45\,/\,40) \\
&= [8\,(40)\,/\,30] \times 1.125 \\
&= [320\,/\,30] \times 1.125 \\
&= 10.67 \times 1.125 \\
&= 12\,/\,min
\end{aligned}
$$

Since the *SWI* is greater than 11 / min, it does not indicate a successful weaning outcome.

**EXERCISE**

The following parameters and measurements are collected during mechanical ventilation. Use the data provided and calculate the simplified weaning index. Does this index indicate a successful weaning outcome?

$f_{mv} = 6/min$, PIP = 35 cm $H_2O$, No PEEP used, MIP = –40 cm $H_2O$, $P_aCO_{2mv} = 38$ mm Hg.

**ANSWER**

$SWI = 4.99/min$ or $5/min$.
Since the *SWI* is less than 9/min, it indicates a successful weaning outcome.

**REFERENCES**

Jabour, 1991

## Self-Assessment Questions

83a. With the exception of MIP, all parameters used in the Simplified Weaning Index are measured when the patient is receiving:

(A) spontaneous ventilation

(B) mechanical ventilation

(C) pressure support ventilation (PSV)

(D) synchronized intermittent mandatory ventilation (SIMV)

83b. When the Simplified Weaning Index is less than _____ /min, it is predictive of weaning _____.

(A) 9, success

(B) 9, failure

(C) 11, success

(D) 11, failure

83c. When the Simplified Weaning Index is more than _____ /min, it is predictive of weaning _____.

(A) 9, success

(B) 9, failure

(C) 11, success

(D) 11, failure

83d. Use the following measurements to calculate a patient's Simplified Weaning Index: $f_{mv} = 8/min$, PIP = 33 cm $H_2O$, PEEP = 0 cm $H_2O$, MIP = –38 cm $H_2O$, $P_aCO_{2mv} = 36$ mm Hg. Does this index show a successful weaning outcome?

(A) 5, Yes

(B) 5, No

(C) 6, Yes

(D) 6, No

83e.  Use the following measurements to calculate a patient's Simplified Weaning Index: $f_{mv}$ = 12/min, PIP = 40 cm $H_2O$, PEEP = 5 cm $H_2O$, MIP = –32 cm $H_2O$, $P_aCO_{2mv}$ = 45 mm Hg. Does this index show a successful weaning outcome?

(A) 15, Yes

(B) 15, No

(C) 17, Yes

(D) 17, No

83f.  The following parameters and measurements are collected while providing mechanical ventilation to a patient. Calculate the simplified weaning index. What does this index show in regard to weaning success? $f_{mv}$ = 10/min, PIP = 50 cm $H_2O$, PEEP = 10 cm $H_2O$, MIP = –25 cm $H_2O$, $P_aCO_{2mv}$ = 42 mm Hg.

(A) 13, predictive of weaning success

(B) 13, predictive of weaning failure

(C) 17, predictive of weaning success

(D) 17, predictive of weaning failure

# Basic Statistics

# and Educational Calculations

CHAPTER

# Statistics Terminology

| | |
|---|---|
| *Coefficient of Variation (CV)* | Expresses the standard deviation as a percent of the mean: $$CV = \left(\frac{s}{X}\right) \times 100\%$$ Coefficient of variation ($CV$) is useful in comparing the dispersion of two or more sets of data measured by different instruments or methods. For example, if set $A$ of measurements has a $CV$ of 25% and set $B$ of measurements has a $CV$ of 14%, we can infer that the measuring instrument or method for set $A$ has more random errors than that for set $B$. (See sample calculation in this section.) |
| *Confidence Level* | Probability level. The confidence level is usually set at 95% (0.05 level), which means that there is a 95% probability that the sample population is distributed in the same way as the whole population. For example, if statistical analysis provides a conclusion that is accepted at the 0.05 level, the researcher can be 95% confident that the conclusion can be applied to the whole population. |
| *Control Group* | A group of subjects whose selection and experiences are identical in every way possible to those of the treatment (experimental) group except that they do not receive the treatment. |
| *Control Variable* | A variable in the experimental design that is neutralized or canceled out by the researcher. This is the factor controlled by the researcher to neutralize any undesirable effect that might otherwise distort the observed outcome. |
| *Correlation Coefficient (r)* | Describes the relationship between two interval variables. It ranges from $-1$ (most negative relationship) to $+1$ (most positive relationship). For example, the coefficient may be positively related ($r = 0.86$) as in $F_IO_2$ and $P_aO_2$, or it may be negatively related ($r = -0.77$) as in alveolar ventilation and $P_aCO_2$. If a regression line is constructed from the data points, it can "predict" one interval variable given the other interval variable. |

| | |
|---|---|
| *Cut Score* | The minimal passing score of an objective test or questionnaire. It is determined by a formula using the consensus of a group of subject-matter experts. (See sample calculation in this section.) |
| *Dependent Variable* | A response or output caused by the use of treatment or placebo. This is the factor observed and measured by the researcher to determine the effect of the independent variable. |
| *Hypothesis* | A suggested solution to a problem. It has the following characteristics: (1) It should have a statement based on logical derivation of a conclusion from facts; (2) it should be stated clearly and concisely in the form of a declarative sentence; and (3) it should be testable. |
| *Independent Variable* | A variable or input that operates within a person or within his or her surroundings that affects behavior or outcome. This is the factor selected and manipulated by the researcher to determine the relationship to an observed outcome. |
| *Interval Scale* | Lists the order of data and sets the interval or distance between measurements. For example, patient 1's heart rate is 120/min while patient 2's heart rate is 100/min. Not only is the first patient's heart rate higher than the second patient's, but also it is 20 bears higher. |

*Kuder–Richardson Reliability Coefficient (K-R21)*

A test reliability formula that is equivalent to the average of all possible split-half reliability coefficients. (See sample calculation in this section.)

$$K\text{-}R21 = 1 - \frac{\overline{X}(n - \overline{X})}{ns^2}$$

K-R21 = Kuder-Richardson reliability coefficient, Formula 21
$\overline{X}$ = Mean score on the test
$n$ = Number of items in the test
$s^2$ = Test variance

| | |
|---|---|
| *Likert Scale* | A five-point scale in which the intervals between successive measurements are to be equal. The Likert scale is often used in questionnaires since it can easily record the extent of agreement or disagreement with a statement. |
| *Mean* | The average measurement. It is computed by adding all measurements and then dividing by the number of measurements. (See sample calculation in this section.) |
| *Median* | The measurement in the middle of a ranked distribution; 50% of the measurements fall above it, and the other 50% fall below it. (See sample calculation in this section.) |

| | |
|---|---|
| *Mode* | The most frequently occurring measurement in a ranked distribution. If two measurements share the highest frequency count, the ranked distribution is called bimodal. (See example in this section.) |
| *Nominal Scale* | The term "nominal" means "to name." A nominal scale classifies data into categories with no relation existing between the categories. For example, three categories of disease: chronic obstructive pulmonary disease, 1; congestive heart failure, 2; cystic fibrosis, 3. |
| *Null Hypothesis* | A negative or "no differences" version of a hypothesis. When a null hypothesis is rejected, a significant difference between the two means is said to have occurred in a research study. (See *t*-test in this section.) |
| *Ordinal Scale* | The term "ordinal" means "to rank in order." An ordinal scale ranks data in terms of more than or less than. For example, no cyanosis, mild cyanosis, moderate cyanosis, severe cyanosis. |
| *Placebo* | An inert substance given to the control group in the same manner as to the treatment group. Placebos are often used in medical research to make it impossible for the subjects to determine whether or not they are receiving the active substance under study. |
| *Range* | The distance or measurement between the lowest and highest measurements. (See example in this section.) |
| *Rating Scale* | A device that can be used to summarize the observed activity. This scale may have three, five, seven, or an infinite number of points on a line with descriptive statements on both ends. |
| *Ratio Scale* | Data of physical science measurements including a true zero value such as blood pressure, arterial $PO_2$, height, and weight. |
| *Reliability* | Consistency. A *reliable* research study yields *consistent* results when the study is repeated. Reliability ranges from 0% (least reliable) to 100% (most reliable). |

*Revised Nedelsky Procedure*

A three-step procedure to calculate the Cut Score of an evaluation instrument such as a multiple-choice exam. (See sample calculations in this section.)

*Spearman-Brown Formula*   A formula to calculate the whole test reliability ($r_2$). (See sample calculation in this section.)

$$r_2 = \frac{n(r_1)}{1 + (n-1)r_1}$$

$r_2$ = whole test reliability

$n$ = number of parts (for halves, $n = 2$)

$r_1$ = correlation coefficient

*Split-Half Reliability*

A reliability index of the internal consistency of a test that enables a researcher to determine whether the halves of a test are measuring the same quality or characteristic. The test is divided into halves, usually the odd-numbered items and the even-numbered items.

The correlation coefficient ($r_1$) is calculated by using the scores obtained by all students on one half of the exam and those obtained on the other half of the same exam. For a group of 30 students, 30 pairs of scores (30 scores for odd-numbered items and 30 scores for even-numbered items) would be used to calculate the correlation coefficient ($r_1$).

From the correlation coefficient ($r_1$), the whole test reliability ($r_2$) can be calculated by the Spearman-Brown formula.

*Standard Deviation (s)*

A measure of the spread or dispersion of a distribution of measurements. $N - 1$ in the equation is the degree of freedom. (See sample calculation in this section.) (In text, the abbreviation for standard deviation is SD.)

In the blood gas laboratory, standard deviation is used along with the mean to create a Levey-Jennings chart for graphic illustration of quality control results. Results falling within two standard deviations ($\pm 2$ SD) from the mean are considered "in control." Results falling outside two standard deviations from the mean are considered "out of control," and corrective actions must be taken to bring the results within two standard deviations.

*Standard (z) Scores*

A standard ($z$) score reflects the distance (in terms of standard deviations) of a measurement away from the mean. A $z$ score of $+ 1.5$ means that the measurement is 1.5 standard deviations *above* the mean. A $z$ score of $- 1.5$ means that the measurement is 1.5 standard deviations *below* the mean. (See sample calculation in this section.)

*t-test*

The *t*-test allows a researcher to compare two means to determine the probability that the difference between the means is a real difference rather than a chance difference.

If the calculated $t$ value is greater than the table $t$ value at a specific confidence ($p$) level, then then null hypothesis (i.e., that the means are equal) can be rejected at the $p$ level. In other words, there is a statistical difference between the two means.

If the calculated $t$ value is smaller than the table $t$ value, there is no statistical difference between the means.

*Treatment Group*

A group of subjects whose selection and experiences are identical in every way possible to those of the control group. This is the group that receives the treatment.

| *Validity* | The precision with which a research study measures what it purports to measure. |
|---|---|
| *Variance ($s^2$)* | The square of the standard deviation. (See example calculation in this section.) |

**REFERENCES**   Chatburn; Gross; Nedelsky; Tuckman; White

# Measures of Central Tendency

**EXAMPLES 1-8**

Ten scores from a 100-item final exam are ranked and listed as follows: 66, 66, 66, 73, 75, 79, 82, 84, 87, and 87. For examples 1 through 8, write or calculate the (1) range, (2) mode, (3) mean, (4) median, (5) standard deviation, (6) variance, (7) coefficient of variation, and (8) standard scores for 73 points and 82 points on the exam.

**SOLUTION 1**

*Range*: The range for the 10 exam scores is 66 to 87 points (21 points).

**SOLUTION 2**

*Mode*: The most frequently occurring measurement of these 10 exam scores is 66 points.

**SOLUTION 3**

*Mean* ($\overline{X}$):

$$\overline{X} = \frac{Sum\ of\ exam\ scores}{Number\ of\ scores}$$

$$= \frac{66 + 66 + 66 + 73 + 75 + 79 + 82 + 84 + 87 + 87}{10}$$

$$= \frac{765}{10}$$

$$= 76.5\ points$$

**SOLUTION 4**

*Median*: Since median is the measurement in the middle of this ranked 10-number distribution, it falls between 75 (the fifth number) and 79 (the sixth number). The median is therefore $\frac{75 + 79}{2} = \frac{154}{2} = 77$ points.

## SOLUTION 5

*Standard Deviation (s):*

| Value of $X$ | Mean ($\overline{X}$) | $(X - \overline{X})$ | $(X - \overline{X})^2$ |
|---|---|---|---|
| 66 | 76.5 | $-10.5$ | 110.25 |
| 66 | 76.5 | $-10.5$ | 110.25 |
| 66 | 76.5 | $-10.5$ | 110.25 |
| 73 | 76.5 | $-3.5$ | 12.25 |
| 75 | 76.5 | $-1.5$ | 2.25 |
| 79 | 76.5 | 2.5 | 6.25 |
| 82 | 76.5 | 5.5 | 30.25 |
| 84 | 76.5 | 7.5 | 56.25 |
| 87 | 76.5 | 10.5 | 110.25 |
| 87 | 76.5 | 10.5 | 110.25 |
| | | 0 | 658.50 |

$$
\begin{aligned}
s &= \frac{\sqrt{\text{Sum of }(X - \overline{X})^2}}{\text{Degree of freedom}} \\[2mm]
&= \frac{\sqrt{\text{Sum of }(X - \overline{X})^2}}{(\text{Number of scores} - 1)} \\[2mm]
&= \frac{\sqrt{\text{Sum of }(X - \overline{X})^2}}{(N - 1)} \\[2mm]
&= \sqrt{\frac{658.5}{(10 - 1)}} \\[2mm]
&= \sqrt{\frac{658.5}{9}} \\[2mm]
&= \sqrt{73.17} \\[2mm]
&= 8.554 \text{ points}
\end{aligned}
$$

## SOLUTION 6

*Variance ($s^2$):* Since variance is the square of the standard deviation, it is 73.17 ($8.554^2$).

## SOLUTION 7

*Coefficient of Variation (CV):*

$$
\begin{aligned}
CV &= \left(\frac{\text{standard deviation}}{\text{mean}}\right) \times 100\% \\[2mm]
&= \left(\frac{s}{\overline{X}}\right) \times 100\% \\[2mm]
&= \left(\frac{8.554}{76.5}\right) \times 100\% \\[2mm]
&= 0.1118 \times 100\% \\[2mm]
&= 11.18\%
\end{aligned}
$$

## SOLUTION 8

*Standard (z) Scores:* For a score of 73 points on the exam, the standard score (z) is calculated as follows:

$$
\begin{aligned}
z &= \frac{X - \overline{X}}{s} \\[2mm]
&= \frac{73 - 76.5}{8.554} \\[2mm]
&= \frac{-3.5}{8.554} \\[2mm]
&= -0.41
\end{aligned}
$$

The z score for 73 is 0.41 standard deviation *below* the mean.

For a score of 82 points on the exam, the standard score ($z$) is calculated as follows:

$$z = \frac{X - \overline{X}}{s}$$

$$= \frac{82 - 76.5}{8.554}$$

$$= \frac{5.5}{8.554}$$

$$= 0.64$$

The $z$ score for 82 is 0.64 standard deviation *above* the mean.

## EXAMPLE 9

The mean and one standard deviation for a series of $PO_2$ calibration measurements are 157 mm Hg and ±3 mm Hg, respectively. If two standard deviations from the mean are used to set the limit of acceptance, which of the following six $PO_2$ calibration points is out of range? 155, 160, 153, 157, 164, 163 mm Hg.

## SOLUTION 9

164 mm Hg is out of range.

A mean $PO_2$ of 157 mm Hg with one standard deviation (SD) of ±3 mm Hg would have two SD of ±6 mm Hg. Therefore, the acceptable range for $PO_2$ calibration is 151 (157 − 6) mm Hg to 163 (157 + 6) mm Hg. Of the six calibration points, 164 mm Hg is the only one outside this acceptable range.

## EXAMPLE 10

The mean and one standard deviation for a series of normal pH calibration measurements are 7.375 and ±0.002, respectively. If measurements falling within two standard deviations from the mean are considered acceptable, which of the following seven pH calibration points is out of range? 7.379, 7.376, 7.374, 7.377, 7.370, 7.375, and 7.376.

## SOLUTION 10

7.370 is out of range.

A mean pH of 7.375 with one standard deviation (SD) of ±0.002 would have two SD of ±0.004. The acceptable range for pH calibration is therefore 7.371 (7.375 − 0.004) to 7.379 (7.375 + 0.004). Of the seven calibration points, 7.370 is the only one outside this acceptable range.

# Exercises

**EXERCISE 1-8**

Nine mixed-venous oxygen content ($C\bar{v}O_2$) measurements in volume percent (vol%), are ranked and listed as follows: 12, 14, 14, 15, 15, 16, 16, 16, and 17. Write or calculate the (1) range, (2) mode, (3) mean, (4) median, (5) standard deviation, (6) variance, (7) coefficient of variation, and (8) standard scores for 12 vol% and 16 vol%.

**SOLUTION 1**

*Range:* The range for the nine $C\bar{v}O_2$ measurements is 12 to 17 vol% (5 vol%).

**SOLUTION 2**

*Mode:* The most frequently occurring measurement of these nine $C\bar{v}O_2$ values is 16 vol%.

**SOLUTION 3**

*Mean ($\overline{X}$):*

$$\overline{X} = \frac{\text{Sum of } C\bar{v}O_2 \text{ measurements}}{\text{Number of measurements}}$$

$$= \frac{12 + 14 + 14 + 15 + 15 + 16 + 16 + 16 + 17}{9}$$

$$= \frac{135}{9}$$

$$= 15 \text{ vol\%}$$

**SOLUTION 4**

*Median:* Rank the nine numbers as follows:
12, 14, 14, 15, 15, 16, 16, 16, 17.
Since median is the measurement in the middle of this ranked nine-number distribution, it falls between the fourth number and the sixth number. The median is therefore 15 vol%—the second 15 having four numbers before it and four numbers behind it.

## SOLUTION 5

*Standard Deviation (s):*

| Value of X | Mean ($\overline{X}$) | ($X - \overline{X}$) | ($X - \overline{X}$)² |
|---|---|---|---|
| 12 | 1.5 | −3 | 9 |
| 14 | 1.5 | −1 | 1 |
| 14 | 1.5 | −1 | 1 |
| 15 | 1.5 | 0 | 0 |
| 15 | 1.5 | 0 | 0 |
| 16 | 1.5 | 1 | 1 |
| 16 | 1.5 | 1 | 1 |
| 16 | 1.5 | 1 | 1 |
| 17 | 1.5 | 2 | 4 |
| | | 0 | 18 |

$$
\begin{aligned}
s &= \sqrt{\frac{\text{Sum of } (X - \overline{X})^2}{\text{Degree of freedom}}} \\[1mm]
&= \sqrt{\frac{\text{Sum of } (X - \overline{X})^2}{(\text{Number of } C_{\overline{v}}O_2 \text{ measurements} - 1)}} \\[1mm]
&= \sqrt{\frac{\text{Sum of } (X - \overline{X})^2}{(N - 1)}} \\[1mm]
&= \sqrt{\frac{18}{(9 - 1)}} \\[1mm]
&= \sqrt{\frac{18}{8}} \\[1mm]
&= \sqrt{2.25} \\[1mm]
&= 1.5 \text{ vol\%}
\end{aligned}
$$

## SOLUTION 6

*Variance ($s^2$):* Since variance is the square of the standard deviation, it is therefore 2.25 ($1.5^2$).

## SOLUTION 7

*Coefficient of Variation (CV):*

$$
\begin{aligned}
CV &= \left(\frac{\text{standard deviation}}{\text{mean}}\right) \times 100\% \\[1mm]
&= \left(\frac{s}{\overline{X}}\right) \times 100\% \\[1mm]
&= \left(\frac{1.5}{15}\right) \times 100\% \\[1mm]
&= 0.1 \times 100\% \\[1mm]
&= 10\%
\end{aligned}
$$

## SOLUTION 8

*Standard (z) Scores:* For 12 vol%, the standard score (z) is calculated as follows:

$$
\begin{aligned}
z &= \frac{X - \overline{X}}{s} \\[1mm]
&= \frac{12 - 15}{1.5} \\[1mm]
&= \frac{-3}{1.5} \\[1mm]
&= -2
\end{aligned}
$$

The z score for 12 vol% is 2 standard deviation *below* the mean.

For a score of 16, the standard score ($z$) is calculated as follows:

$$z = \frac{X - \overline{X}}{s}$$

$$= \frac{16 - 15}{1.5}$$

$$= \frac{1}{1.5}$$

$$= 0.67$$

The $z$ score for 16 vol% is 0.67 standard deviation *above* the mean.

## EXAMPLE 9

The mean and one standard deviation for a series of $PO_2$ calibration measurements are 102 mm Hg and ±1 mm Hg, respectively. If two standard deviations from the mean are used to set the limit of acceptance, which of the following five $PO_2$ calibration points is out of range? 102, 103, 99, 104, and 100 mm Hg.

## SOLUTION 9

99 mm Hg is out of range.

A mean $PO_2$ of 102 mm Hg with one standard deviation (SD) of ±1 mm Hg would have two SD of ±2 mm Hg. Therefore, the acceptable range for $PO_2$ calibration is 100 (102 − 2) mm Hg to 104 (102 + 2) mm Hg. Of the five calibration points, 99 mm Hg is the only one outside this acceptable range.

## EXAMPLE 10

The mean and one standard deviation for a series of acidotic pH calibration measurements are 7.135 and ±0.015, respectively. If measurements falling within two standard deviations from the mean are considered acceptable, which of the following six pH calibration points is out of range? 7.137, 7.165, 7.175, 7.125, 7.106, and 7.135.

## SOLUTION 10

7.175 is out of range.

A mean pH of 7.135 with one standard deviation (SD) of ±0.015 would have two SD of ±0.030. The acceptable range for pH calibration is therefore 7.105 (7.135 − 0.030) to 7.165 (7.135 + 0.030). Of the six calibration points, 7.175 is the only one outside this acceptable range.

## EXERCISE 11

The mean and one standard deviation for a series of $PCO_2$ calibration measurements are 44.9 mm Hg and ±0.5 mm Hg, respectively. Which of the following five $PCO_2$ calibration points (44.0, 45.6, 43.5, 45.0, and 46.5 mm Hg) is out of range if (A) *two* standard deviations from the mean are used to set the limit of acceptance; (B) *three* standard deviations from the mean are used to set the limit of acceptance.

**SOLUTION 11**

(A) 43.5 and 46.5 mm Hg are out of range; (B) 46.5 mm Hg is out of range.

(A) A mean $PCO_2$ of 44.9 mm Hg with one standard deviation (SD) of ±0.5 mm Hg would have two SD of ±1.0 mm Hg. Therefore, the acceptable range for $PCO_2$ calibration is 43.9 (44.9 − 1.0) mm Hg to 45.9 (44.9 + 1.0) mm Hg. Of the five calibration points, 43.5 mm Hg and 46.5 mm Hg are the $PCO_2$ measurements outside this acceptable range.

(B) If three standard deviations (±1.5 mm Hg) were used, the acceptable range for $PCO_2$ calibration would become 43.4 (44.9 − 1.5) mm Hg to 46.4 (44.9 + 1.5) mm Hg. Of the five calibration points, 46.5 mm Hg is the $PCO_2$ outside this acceptable range.

# Test Reliability

## Kuder-Richardson Reliability Coefficient (K-R21)

The Kuder-Richardson reliability coefficient calculates the test reliability when the following are known: (1) mean score of the test, (2) variance of the test, and (3) number of items in the test.
The reliability coefficient ranges from 0 (least reliable) to 1 (most reliable).

**EXAMPLE**

Ten scores from a 100-item final exam are ranked and listed as follows: 66, 66, 66, 73, 75, 79, 72, 84, 87, and 87. Calculate the reliability index of this exam using the Kuder-Richardson reliability coefficient (K-R21) formula. From previous examples, the mean (Example 3) and variance (Example 6) have been calculated and obtained. The reliability index may be calculated as follows:

$\overline{X}$ (mean score)  = 76.5

$n$ (number of items in the test) =  100

$s^2$ (variance)  = 73.17

$$\text{K-R21} = 1 - \frac{\overline{X}(n - \overline{X})}{ns^2}$$

$$= 1 - \frac{76.5(100 - 76.5)}{100(73.17)}$$

$$= 1 - \frac{76.5(23.5)}{7317}$$

$$= 1 - \frac{1797.75}{7317}$$

$$= 1 - 0.2457$$

$$= 0.7543 \text{ or } 75.43\%$$

The test reliability based on the K-R21 formula is 75.43%.

**EXERCISE 1**

The mean score and variance of a 90-item exam are 72.8 and 66.2, respectively. Calculate the reliability of this exam using the Kuder-Richardson reliability coefficient (K-R21) formula.

## SOLUTION 1

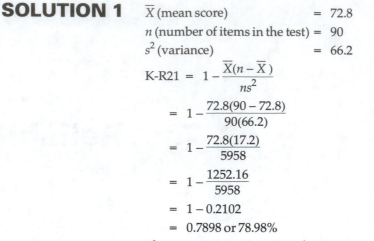

$\overline{X}$ (mean score) = 72.8
$n$ (number of items in the test) = 90
$s^2$ (variance) = 66.2

$$\text{K-R21} = 1 - \frac{\overline{X}(n - \overline{X})}{ns^2}$$

$$= 1 - \frac{72.8(90 - 72.8)}{90(66.2)}$$

$$= 1 - \frac{72.8(17.2)}{5958}$$

$$= 1 - \frac{1252.16}{5958}$$

$$= 1 - 0.2102$$

$$= 0.7898 \text{ or } 78.98\%$$

The test reliability based on the K-R21 formula is 78.98%.

## EXERCISE 2

On a standardized 160-item comprehensive exam, the mean score and variance are 129.3 and 110.8, respectively. Use the Kuder–Richardson reliability coefficient (K-R21) formula to calculate the reliability of this exam.

## SOLUTION 2

$\overline{X}$ (mean score) = 129.3
$n$ (number of items in the test) = 160
$s^2$ (variance) = 110.8

$$\text{K-R21} = 1 - \frac{\overline{X}(n - \overline{X})}{ns^2}$$

$$= 1 - \frac{129.3(160 - 129.3)}{160(110.8)}$$

$$= 1 - \frac{129.3(30.7)}{17728}$$

$$= 1 - \frac{3969.51}{17728}$$

$$= 1 - 0.2239$$

$$= 0.7761 \text{ or } 77.61\%$$

The test reliability based on the K-R21 formula is 77.61%.

## SPEARMAN–BROWN FORMULA

The Spearman-Brown Formula calculates the whole test reliability when the correlation coefficient of the split-half scores is known. The split-half technique separates the exam into two halves, usually the odd-numbered and even-numbered exam items. Pairs of scores from the exam are then used to calculate the correlation coefficient.

The whole test reliability index ranges from 0 (least reliable) to 1 (most reliable).

## EXAMPLE

On a 60-item exam, the scores obtained by each student on the odd-numbered items and the even-numbered items are compared. The correlation coefficient ($r_1$) of the split-half technique is 0.67 for the entire class of 28 students (28 pairs of scores). Based on the information given, calculate the whole test reliability ($r_2$) with the Spearman-Brown formula.

$r_2$ : whole test reliability

$n$ (number of parts; for halves, $n = 2$) = 2

$r_1$ (correlation coefficient) = 0.67

$$r_2 = \frac{n(r_1)}{1 + (n-1)r_1}$$

$$= \frac{2(0.67)}{1 + (2-1)0.67}$$

$$= \frac{1.34}{1 + (1)0.67}$$

$$= \frac{1.34}{1 + 0.67}$$

$$= \frac{1.34}{1.67}$$

$$= 0.8024 \text{ or } 80.24\%$$

The whole test reliability based on the Spearman–Brown formula is 80.24%.

## EXERCISE 1

A 90-item exam was given to a class of 34 students. Thirty-four pairs of scores were obtained by splitting and scoring the exam by odd-numbered and even-numbered items. The correlation coefficient ($r_1$) for the 34 pairs of scores by this split-half technique is 0.58.

Based on the information given, calculate the whole test reliability ($r_2$) with the Spearman-Brown formula.

$r_2$ : whole test reliability

$n$ (number of parts; for halves, $n = 2$) = 2

$r_1$ (correlation coefficient) = 0.58

$$r_2 = \frac{n(r_1)}{1 + (n-1)r_1}$$

$$= \frac{2(0.58)}{1 + (2-1)0.58}$$

$$= \frac{1.16}{1 + (1)0.58}$$

$$= \frac{1.16}{1 + 0.58}$$

$$= \frac{1.16}{1.58}$$

$$= 0.7342 \text{ or } 73.42\%$$

The whole test reliability based on the Spearman-Brown formula is 73.42%.

## EXERCISE 2

Twenty pairs of scores are recorded from a 60-item exam administered to a class of 20 students. Each pair of scores represents the number of correct answers obtained by each student from the odd-numbered and even-numbered exam items. The correlation coefficient ($r_1$) for the 20 pairs of scores is 0.75.

Based on the information given, what is the calculated whole test reliability ($r_2$) with the Spearman-Brown formula?

## SOLUTION 2

$r_2$ : whole test reliability

$n$ (number of parts; for halves, $n = 2$) = 2

$r_1$ (correlation coefficient) = 0.75

$$r_2 = \frac{n(r_1)}{1 + (n-1)r_1}$$

$$= \frac{2(0.75)}{1 + (2-1)0.75}$$

$$= \frac{1.5}{1 + (1)0.75}$$

$$= \frac{1.5}{1 + 0.75}$$

$$= \frac{1.5}{1.75}$$

$$= 0.8571 \text{ or } 85.71\%$$

The whole test reliability based on the Spearman-Brown formula is 85.71%.

# Cut Score: Revised Nedelsky Procedure

In 1954, Leo Nedelsky published a procedure to compute the cut score (minimum passing score) of a multiple-choice exam. Among other factors that make an exam item "difficult" or "easy," the Nedelsky procedure accounts for the degree of difficulty of the distractors in a multiple-choice exam item.

The original procedure was revised by Leon J. Gross in 1985. In this revised procedure, a three-point (0 to 2) distribution is used. The revised procedure by Gross is summarized as follows.

## STEP 1

All responses to a multiple-choice exam item are evaluated by a group of subject-matter experts. Consensus is then obtained from these experts, and points ranging from 0 to 2 are assigned to each response.

The one *correct response* is scored *2 points* (weight of correct response).

Each *plausible but incorrect response* is scored *1 point* (weight of plausible, incorrect response). This represents an "acceptable" error for the minimally competent examinee.

Each *implausible and incorrect response* is scored *0 points* (weight of implausible, incorrect response). This represents an unacceptable error that should have been avoided even by the minimally competent examinee.

## STEP 2

The minimal pass index (MPI) for each exam item is calculated by:

$$MPI = \frac{\text{Weight of correct response}}{\text{Sum of all weights for each item}}$$

## STEP 3

Cut score  =  MPI of all exam items  ×  95%

A value of 95% is used to avoid extreme cut scores in the original Nedelsky procedure. This value may be adjusted up or down depending on the degree of chance and perfection (number of responses) in each exam item.

**EXAMPLE 1**   Find the minimal pass index (MPI) of the multiple-choice exam item below.

Under normal tidal volume and respiratory rate, the $F_IO_2$ provided by a nasal cannula at 2 L/min of oxygen is about

A. 21%

B. 24%

C. 28%

D. 32%

**STEP 1**   The four responses are evaluated by a group of experts. Their consensus and point assignments to each response are as follows.

A. 21%:   0 points

B. 24%:   1 point

C. 28%:   2 points

D. 32%:   1 point

Response (A) is scored 0 points because even the minimally competent examinee should be able to eliminate this option since the $F_IO_2$ provided by a nasal cannula at 2 L/min of oxygen must be greater than 21% ($F_IO_2$ of room air).

Responses (B) and (D) are score 1 point each because they are incorrect but plausible responses.

Response (C) is scored 2 points because it is the correct response.

**STEP 2**   The minimal pass index (MPI) of this exam item is therefore:

$$MPI = \frac{\text{Weight of correct response}}{\text{Sum of all weights for item}}$$

$$= \frac{2 \text{ points}}{(0 + 1 + 2 + 1) \text{ points}}$$

$$= \frac{2}{4}$$

$$= 0.5$$

**EXAMPLE 2**   Calculate the cut score of a 10-item multiple-choice exam with the following minimal pass indices (MPI) for the 10 exam items: 0.67, 0.5, 1.0, 0.67, 0.4, 0.5, 0.4, 0.67, 0.5, and 1.0.

Cut score =  MPI of all exam items × 95%

$$= (0.67+0.5+1.0+0.67+0.4+0.5+0.4+0.67+0.5+1.0)$$
$$\times 95\%$$

$$= 6.31 \times 95\%$$

$$= 5.99 \text{ or } 6 \text{ points}$$

The cut score (minimal passing score) of this 10-item multiple-choice exam is 6 points.

**EXERCISE 1**

As shown below, the point assignments for each response to an exam item are provided by a group of experts. What is the minimal pass index (MPI) of this exam item?

The preferred puncture site for arterial blood gas sampling in an adult is the

A.  radial artery:        2 points
B.  umbilical artery:     0 points
C.  brachial artery:      1 point
D.  coronary artery:      0 points

**SOLUTION 1**

$$\text{MPI} = \frac{\text{Weight of correct response}}{\text{Sum of all weights for item}}$$

$$= \frac{2 \text{ points}}{3 \text{ points}}$$

$$= 0.67$$

**EXERCISE 2**

Use the revised Nedelsky procedure to calculate the cut score of a nine-item multiple-choice exam with the following minimal pass indices for the nine exam items: 0.5, 1.0, 0.67, 0.4, 0.4, 0.67, 0.5, 0.67, and 0.4.

**SOLUTION 2**

Cut score = MPI of all exam items $\times$ 95%

= (0.5+1.0+0.67+0.4+0.4+0.67+0.5+0.67+0.4) $\times$ 95%

= 5.21 $\times$ 95%

= 4.95 or 5 points

**EXERCISE 3**

If the sum of all minimal pass indices (MPI) in a 98-item multiple-choice exam is 81, what is the cut score using the revised Nedelsky procedure?

**SOLUTION 3**

Cut score = MPI of all exam items $\times$ 95%

= 81 $\times$ 95%

= 76.95 or 77 points

**REFERENCES**

Gross; Nedelsky

# 4

# Answer Key

# to Self-Assessment Questions

| Question no. | Answer | Question No. | Answer |
| --- | --- | --- | --- |
| 1a | (B) | 13d | (B) |
| 1b | (A) | 13e | (C) |
| | | | |
| 2a | (D) | 14a | (A) |
| 2b | (D) | 14b | (B) |
| 2c | (C) | 14c | (E) |
| 2d | (B) | 14d | (D) |
| | | | |
| 3a | (A) | 15a | (E) |
| 3b | (D) | 15b | (B) |
| 3c | (C) | 15c | (B) |
| 3d | (D) | | |
| | | 16a | (D) |
| 4a | (C) | 16b | (C) |
| 4b | (D) | 16c | (D) |
| 4c | (B) | 16d | (C) |
| | | 16e | (E) |
| 5a | (A) | 16f | (B) |
| 5b | (B) | 16g | (A) |
| | | | |
| 6a | (D) | 17a | (A) |
| 6b | (A) | 17b | (D) |
| 6c | (D) | 17c | (E) |
| | | | |
| 7a | (E) | 18a | (C) |
| 7b | (C) | 18b | (A) |
| | | 18c | (E) |
| 8a | (C) | 18d | (D) |
| 8b | (B) | 18e | (C) |
| 8c | (E) | 18f | (D) |
| | | 18g | (A) |
| 9a | (C) | | |
| 9b | (A) | 19a | (C) |
| | | 19b | (A) |
| 10a | (C) | 19c | (D) |
| 10b | (B) | 19d | (A) |
| 10c | (A) | 19e | (E) |
| 10d | (A) | | |
| 10e | (C) | 20a | (B) |
| 10f | (E) | 20b | (D) |
| | | 20c | (A) |
| 11a | (E) | 20d | (B) |
| 11b | (D) | | |
| 11c | (A) | 21a | (E) |
| 11d | (E) | 21b | (C) |
| | | 21c | (D) |
| 12a | (C) | 21d | (B) |
| 12b | (C) | 21e | (C) |
| 12c | (D) | | |
| 12d | (D) | 22a | (C) |
| | | 22b | (A) |
| 13a | (A) | 22c | (C) |
| 13b | (D) | 22d | (E) |
| 13c | (B) | 22e | (D) |

| Question no. | Answer | Question no. | Answer |
|---|---|---|---|
| 22f | (C) | 30d | (D) |
| 22g | (D) | 30e | (B) |
| 22h | (B) | | |
| 22i | (E) | 31a | (C) |
| 22j | (C) | 31b | (A) |
| 22k | (D) | 31c | (A) |
| 22l | (C) | | |
| 22m | (E) | 32a | (D) |
| | | 32b | (C) |
| 23a | (C) | | |
| 23b | (C) | 33a | (E) |
| 23c | (B) | 33b | (C) |
| 23d | (C) | 33c | (C) |
| 23e | (E) | | |
| 23f | (D) | 34a | $FEV_1 = 0.75$ L, FVC = 3.5 L, $FEV_{1\%} = 21.4\%$, $FEV_{1\%}$ is abnormal. |
| 23g | (B) | | |
| 23h | (B) | | |
| 23i | (C) | 34b | $FEV_2 = 2.15$ L, FVC = 4.5 L, $FEV_{2\%} = 47.8\%$, $FEV_{2\%}$ is abnormal |
| 23j | (D) | | |
| 23k | (D) | | |
| 23l | (C) | 34c | $FEV_3 = 4.0$ L, FVC = 5.5 L, $FEV_{3\%} = 72.7\%$, $FEV_{3\%}$ is abnormal |
| 23m | (E) | | |
| 24a | (B) | | |
| 24b | (C) | 35a | $FEF_{200\text{-}1200} = 0.6$ L/sec |
| 24c | (C) | 35b | $FEF_{200\text{-}1200} = 1.1$ L/sec |
| 24d | (A) | 35c | $FEF_{200\text{-}1200} = 1.8$ L/sec |
| 25a | (A) | 36a | $FEF_{25\text{-}75\%} = 0.5$ L/sec |
| 25b | (E) | 36b | $FEF_{25\text{-}75\%} = 0.75$ L/sec |
| 25c | (C) | 36c | $FEF_{25\text{-}75\%} = 1.15$ L/sec |
| 26a | (D) | 37a | (D) |
| 26b | (C) | 37b | (C) |
| 26c | (A) | 37c | (A) |
| 26d | (E) | 37d | (C) |
| | | 37e | (C) |
| 27a | (A) | 37f | (B) |
| 27b | (C) | 37g | (C) |
| | | 37h | (B) |
| 28a | (D) | 37i | (C) |
| 28b | (D) | 37j | (C) |
| 28c | (D) | | |
| 28d | (B) | 38a | (D) |
| | | 38b | (A) |
| 29a | (D) | 38c | (D) |
| 29b | (E) | 38d | (E) |
| 29c | (A) | | |
| 29d | (B) | 39a | (C) |
| 29e | (D) | 39b | (A) |
| | | 39c | (E) |
| 30a | (E) | | |
| 30b | (C) | 40a | (D) |
| 30c | (B) | 40b | (C) |

| Question no. | Answer | Question no. | Answer |
| --- | --- | --- | --- |
| 40c | (E) | 45a | (A) |
| 40d | (B) | 45b | (C) |
|  |  | 45c | (B) |
| 41a | (B) | 45d | (D) |
| 41b | (A) | 45e | (B) |
|  |  | 45f | (C) |
| 42a | (C) | 45g | (C) |
| 42b | (C) |  |  |
| 42c | (A) | 46a | (B) |
| 42d | (D) | 46b | (D) |
| 42e | (A) | 46c | (C) |
| 42f | (A) |  |  |
| 42g | (E) | 47a | (B) |
| 42h | (D) | 47b | (D) |
| 42i | (C) | 47c | (C) |
| 42j | (A) | 47d | (A) |
| 42k | (B) | 47e | (C) |
| 42l | (C) | 47f | (D) |
| 42m | (B) | 47g | (B) |
| 42n | (D) | 47h | (C) |
| 42o | (A) |  |  |
| 42p | (A) | 48a | (C) |
| 42q | (E) | 48b | (B) |
| 42r | (A) | 48c | (C) |
| 42s | (D) | 48d | (C) |
| 42t | (E) | 48e | (D) |
| 42u | (B) | 48f | (A) |
|  |  | 48g | (B) |
| 43a | (A) | 48h | (D) |
| 43b | (B) |  |  |
| 43c | (B) | 49a | (C) |
| 43d | (C) | 49b | (C) |
|  |  | 49c | (A) |
| 44a | (C) | 49d | (D) |
| 44b | (D) | 49e | (B) |
| 44c | (E) | 49f | (B) |
| 44d | (E) | 49g | (D) |
| 44e | (D) | 49h | (C) |
| 44f | (A) | 49i | (A) |
| 44g | (E) |  |  |
| 44h | (B) | 50a | (D) |
| 44i | (D) | 50b | (D) |
| 44j | (C) | 50c | (B) |
| 44k | (A) |  |  |
| 44l | (E) | 51a | (B) |
| 44m | (E) | 51b | (C) |
| 44n | (D) | 51c | (E) |
| 44o | (D) | 51d | (C) |
| 44p | (C) | 51e | (C) |
| 44q | (A) | 51f | (D) |
| 44r | (C) | 51g | (C) |
| 44s | (B) | 51h | (B) |
| 44t | (B) | 51i | (B) |
|  |  | 51j | (D) |

| Question no. | Answer | Question no. | Answer |
|---|---|---|---|
| 51k | (C) | 58e | (D) |
| 51l | (B) | 58f | (A) |
| 51m | (B) | 58g | (A) |
| | | | |
| 52a | (B) | 59a | (B) |
| 52b | (A) | 59b | (D) |
| 52c | (B) | 59c | (D) |
| 52d | (C) | 59d | (D) |
| 52e | (D) | 59e | (E) |
| 52f | (C) | 59f | (B) |
| 52g | (D) | 59g | (A) |
| | | 59h | (C) |
| 53a | (A) | 59i | (A) |
| 53b | (C) | 59j | (C) |
| 53c | (D) | 59k | (E) |
| 53d | (E) | | |
| 53e | (B) | 60a | (C) |
| 53f | (E) | 60b | (D) |
| 53g | (B) | 60c | (E) |
| | | 60d | (D) |
| 54a | (C) | | |
| 54b | (C) | 61a | (E) |
| 54c | (D) | 61b | (E) |
| 54d | (E) | 61c | (C) |
| 54e | (A) | 61d | (A) |
| 54f | (B) | | |
| 54g | (E) | 62a | (B) |
| 54h | (C) | 62b | (A) |
| 54i | (C) | 62c | (D) |
| 54j | (D) | 62d | (C) |
| 54k | (B) | | |
| 54l | (E) | 63a | (C) |
| | | 63b | (A) |
| 55a | (C) | 63c | (D) |
| 55b | (B) | 63d | (E) |
| 55c | (C) | 63e | (D) |
| 55d | (E) | 63f | (B) |
| 55e | (D) | 63g | (A) |
| | | 63h | (B) |
| 56a | (A) | 63i | (E) |
| 56b | (D) | | |
| 56c | (A) | 64a | (D) |
| 56d | (A) | 64b | (C) |
| | | 64c | (E) |
| 57a | (D) | 64d | (C) |
| 57b | (C) | | |
| 57c | (C) | 65a | (C) |
| 57d | (A) | 65b | (E) |
| 57e | (A) | | |
| | | 66a | (C) |
| 58a | (E) | 66b | (B) |
| 58b | (C) | 66c | (D) |
| 58c | (D) | | |
| 58d | (B) | 67a | (A) |

| Question no. | Answer | Question no. | Answer |
|---|---|---|---|
| 67b | (E) | 75a | (B) |
| 67c | (D) | 75b | (E) |
| 67d | (E) | 75c | (D) |
|  |  | 75d | (C) |
| 68a | (A) | 75e | (B) |
| 68b | (E) |  |  |
| 68c | (B) | 76a | (B) |
| 68d | (B) | 76b | (C) |
| 68e | (A) | 76c | (D) |
| 68f | (C) |  |  |
| 68g | (E) | 77a | (E) |
| 68h | (B) | 77b | (D) |
| 68i | (C) | 77c | (A) |
| 68j | (C) | 77d | (E) |
| 68k | (A) | 77e | (E) |
|  |  |  |  |
| 69a | (D) | 78a | (B) |
| 69b | (C) | 78b | (C) |
| 69c | (B) | 78c | (D) |
| 69d | (E) |  |  |
| 69e | (B) | 79a | (E) |
| 69f | (C) | 79b | (C) |
| 69g | (C) | 79c | (D) |
| 69h | (A) | 79d | (B) |
| 69i | (B) |  |  |
|  |  | 80a | (A) |
| 70a | (A) | 80b | (D) |
| 70b | (E) | 80c | (C) |
|  |  | 80d | (E) |
| 71a | (B) | 80e | (C) |
| 71b | (D) |  |  |
| 71c | (E) | 81a | (C) |
| 71d | (D) | 81b | (B) |
| 71e | (B) | 81c | (C) |
|  |  | 81d | (B) |
| 72a | (B) | 81e | (A) |
| 72b | (D) | 81f | (E) |
| 72c | (C) |  |  |
| 72d | (A) | 82a | (B) |
| 72e | (C) | 82b | (C) |
|  |  | 82c | (C) |
| 73a | (D) | 82d | (A) |
| 73b | (D) | 82e | (D) |
| 73c | (B) | 92f | (A) |
| 73d | (A) | 82g | (C) |
| 73e | (D) | 82h | (B) |
| 73f | (B) | 82i | (B) |
|  |  |  |  |
| 74a | (C) | 83a | (B) |
| 74b | (D) | 83b | (A) |
| 74c | (A) | 83c | (D) |
| 74d | (E) | 83d | (C) |
|  |  | 83e | (B) |
|  |  | 83f | (D) |

# 5

# Symbols and Abbreviations

# Symbols and Abbreviations Commonly Used in Respiratory Physiology

---

### Primary Symbols

| GAS SYMBOLS | BLOOD SYMBOLS |
|---|---|
| $P$ Pressure | $Q$ Blood volume |
| $V$ Gas volume | $\dot{Q}$ Blood flow |
| $\dot{V}$ Gas volume per unit of time, or flow | $C$ Content in blood |
| $F$ Fractional concentration of gas | $S$ Saturation |

---

### Secondary Symbols

| GAS SYMBOLS | BLOOD SYMBOLS |
|---|---|
| I Inspired | a Arterial |
| E Expired | c Capillary |
| A Alveolar | v Venous |
| T Tidal | $\bar{v}$ Mixed venous |
| D Dead space | |

---

From Des Jardins, T.D. *Cardiopulmonary Anatomy and Physiology: Essentials for Respiratory Care,* 3rd ed. Albany, NY: Delmar Publishers, 1998.

# Abbreviations

%: Percent.

%$_g$: Percent of gas in the mixture.

$a$/A ratio: Arterial / alveolar oxygen tension ratio in %.

BD: Base deficit in mEq/L, negative base excess (–BE).

$BP_{systolic}$: Systolic blood pressure in mm Hg.

$BP_{diastolic}$: Diastolic blood pressure in mm Hg.

BSA: Body surface area in $m^2$.

$C$: Compliance in mL/cm $H_2O$ or L/cm $H_2O$.

°C: degree Celsius.

$C_{dyn}$: Dynamic compliance in mL/cm $H_2O$.

$C_{st}$: Static compliance in mL/cm $H_2O$.

$C_aO_2$: Arterial oxygen content in vol%.

Capacity: Maximum amount of water that air can hold at a given temperature in mg/L or mm Hg.

$C(a-\bar{v})O_2$: Arterial–mixed venous oxygen content difference in vol%.

$C_cO_2$: End-capillary oxygen content in vol%.

$CI$: Cardiac index in L/min/$m^2$.

$Cl^-$: Serum chloride concentration in mEq/L.

cm $H_2O$: Centimeters of water, a unit of pressure measurement.

$CO$: Cardiac output in L/min ($\dot{Q}_T$).

$C_{\bar{v}}O_2$: Mixed venous oxygen content in vol%.

$D$: Density of gas in g/L.

dyne·sec/$cm^5$: dyne·second/centimeter$^5$, a vascular resistance unit.

$E$: Elastance in cm $H_2O$/L.

$ERV$: Expiratory reserve volume in mL or L.

Expired $V_T$: Expired tidal volume in mL or L.

°F: degree Fahrenheit.

$FEF_{25-75\%}$: Forced Expiratory Flow of the middle 50% of vital capacity.

$FEF_{200-1200}$: Forced Expiratory Flow of 200 to 1200 mL of vital capacity.

$FEV_t$: Forced Expiratory Volume (timed).

$FEV_{t\%}$: Forced Expiratory Volume (timed percent).

$F_IO_2$: Inspired oxygen concentration in %.

Flow: Flow rate in L/sec.

$FRC$: Functional residual capacity in mL or L.

g: gram.

g·m/beat: gram·meter/beat, a ventricular stroke work unit.

g·m/beat/$m^2$: gram·meter/beat/meter$^2$, a ventricular stroke work index unit.

gmw: Gram molecular weight in g.

$HCO_3^-$:  (1) Serum bicarbonate concentration in mEq/L.

          (2) Sodium bicarbonate needed to correct base deficit, in mEq/L.

$H_2CO_3$:  Carbonate acid in mEq/L.

Hb:  Hemoglobin content in g%.

*HD*:  Humidity deficit in mg/L.

HR:  Heart rate per minute.

*IC*:  Inspiratory capacity in mL or L.

*ID*:  Internal diameter of endotracheal tube in mm.

*I* time:  Inspiratory time in sec.

*IRV*:  Inspiratory reserve volume in mL or L.

°K:  Kelvin.

kg:  Body weight in kilograms

kPa:  International System (SI) unit for pressure (kilopascal); 1 kPa equals 7.5 torr or mm Hg.

L:  Liter.

L/min:  Liters per minute; LPM.

log:  logarithm.

LPM:  Liters per minute; L/min.

*LVSW*:  Left ventricular stroke work in g·m/beat.

*LVSWI*:  Left ventricular stroke work index in g·m/beat/m$^2$.

*MAP*:  Mean arterial pressure in mm Hg.

*MAWP*:  Mean airway pressure in cm $H_2O$.

min:  Minute.

mL:  Milliliter.

mm Hg:  Millimeters of mercury, a unit of pressure measurement (torr); equal to 0.1333 kPa.

$Na^+$:  Serum sodium concentration in mEq/L.

$O_2$:air:  Oxygen:air entrainment ratio.

$O_2$ consumption:  Estimated to be 130 × BSA in mL/min ($\dot{V}O_2$).

*P*:  Pressure in cm $H_2O$ or mm Hg.

$\Delta P$:  Pressure change in cm $H_2O$.

*P̄A*:  Mean pulmonary artery pressure in mm Hg.

*PA*$_{systolic}$:  Systolic pulmonary artery pressure in mm Hg.

$P(A-a)O_2$:  Alveolar–arterial oxygen tension gradient in mm Hg.

$P_aCO_2$:  Arterial carbon dioxide tension in mm Hg.

$P_AO_2$:  Alveolar oxygen tension in mm Hg.

$P_aO_2$:  Arterial oxygen tension in mm Hg.

$P_B$:  Barometric pressure in mm Hg.

*PCWP*:  Pulmonary capillary wedge pressure in mm Hg.

$P_{\bar{E}}CO_2$:  Mixed expired carbon dioxide tension in mm Hg.

PEEP:  Positive end-expiratory pressure in cm $H_2O$.

$P_g$:  Partial pressure of a dry gas.

pH:  Puissance hydrogen, negative logarithm of $H^+$ ion concentration.

$PH_2O$:  Water vapor pressure, 47 mm Hg saturated at 37 °C.

PIP:  Peak inspiratory pressure in cm $H_2O$.

$P_{max}$:  Maximum airway pressure in cm $H_2O$ (peak airway pressure).

psig:  Pounds per square inch, a gauge pressure.

$P_{st}$:  Static airway pressure in cm $H_2O$ (plateau airway pressure).

$P_{\bar{v}}O_2$:  Mixed venous oxygen tension in mm Hg.

*PVR*: Pulmonary vascular resistance in dyne·sec/cm$^5$.

$\dot{Q}_{sp}/\dot{Q}_T$: Physiologic shunt to total perfusion ratio in %.

$Q_T$: Total perfusion in L/min; cardiac output (*CO*).

*R*: Resistance in cm $H_2O$/L/sec.

RA: Right atrial pressure in mm Hg.

$\overline{RA}$: Mean right atrial pressure in mm Hg.

$R_{aw}$: Airway resistance in cm $H_2O$/L/sec.

RH: Relative humidity in %.

*RR*: Respiratory rate per minute.

$RR_{mech}$: Mechanical ventilator respiratory rate per minute.

$RR_{spon}$: Patient's spontaneous respiratory rate per minute.

*RSBWI*: Rapid Shallow Breathing Weaning Index.

*RV*: Residual volume in mL or L.

*RVSW*: Right ventricular stroke work in g·m/beat.

*RVSWI*: Right ventricular stroke work index in g·m/beat/m$^2$.

$S_aO_2$: Arterial oxygen saturation in %.

sec: Second.

*SV*: Stroke volume in mL or L.

*SVI*: Stroke volume index in mL/m$^2$.

$S_{\overline{v}}O_2$: Mixed venous oxygen saturation in vol%.

*SVR*: Systemic vascular resistance in dyne·sec/cm$^5$.

*SWI*: Simplified Weaning Index.

*t*: Time constant in seconds.

*TLC*: Total lung capacity.

torr: Unit of pressure measurement (mm Hg); 1 torr equals 0.1333 kPa.

*V*: (1) Volume in mL or L.

    (2) Corrected tidal volume in mL or L.

$\Delta V$: Volume change in mL or L.

$\dot{V}_A$: Alveolar minute ventilation in L.

*VC*: Vital capacity in mL or L.

$V_D$: Deadspace volume in mL or L.

$V_D/V_T$: Deadspace to tidal volume ratio in %.

$\dot{V}_E$: Expired minute ventilation in L.

$\dot{V}O_2$: $O_2$ consumption in mL/min.

$V_T$: Tidal volume in mL or L.

$V_T$ mech: Mechanical ventilator tidal volume in mL.

$V_T$ spon: Patient's spontaneous tidal volume in mL.

Vol%: Volume percent.

Volume$_{ATPS}$: Gas volume saturated with water at ambient (room) temperature and pressure.

Volume$_{BTPS}$: Gas volume saturated with water at body temperature (37 °C) and ambient pressure.

# 6

# Units of Measurement

# Pressure Conversions

| cm H$_2$O | mm Hg | psig | kPa |
|-----------|-------|------|-----|
| 1 | 0.735 | 0.0142 | 0.09806 |
| 1.36 | 1 | 0.0193 | 0.1333 |
| 70.31 | 51.7 | 1 | 6.895 |
| 10.197 | 7.501 | 0.145 | 1 |

**EXAMPLES**

To convert cm H$_2$O to mm Hg, multiply cm H$_2$O by 0.735. For example, a central venous pressure reading of 9 cm H$_2$O is about 6.6 mm Hg ($9 \times 0.735 = 6.615$).

To convert mm Hg to cm H$_2$O, multiply mm Hg by 1.36. For example, sea-level barometric pressure of 760 mm Hg is about 1034 cm H$_2$O ($760 \times 1.36 = 1033.6$).

To convert psig to mm Hg, multiply psig by 51.7. For example, a piped-in oxygen gas source of 50 psig equals 2585 mm Hg ($50 \times 51.7 = 2585$).

# French (Fr) and Millimeter (mm) Conversions

| French (Fr) | Millimeter (mm) |
|-------------|-----------------|
| (4) mm + 2 | 1 |
| 1 | $\dfrac{Fr - 2}{4}$ |

**EXAMPLES**

To convert mm to Fr, multiply mm by 4, then add 2. For example, an endotracheal tube with an internal diameter (*ID*) of 2.5 mm equals 12 Fr [(4) 2.5 + 2 = 10 + 2 = 12].

To convert Fr to mm, subtract 2 from Fr, then divide by 4. For example, an 8-Fr suction catheter equals 1.5 mm:

$$\left( \frac{8 - 2}{4} = \frac{6}{4} = 1.5 \right).$$

# Conversions of Conventional and Système International (SI) Units

| MEASUREMENT | CONVENTIONAL UNIT | SI UNIT | CONVERSION FACTOR |
|---|---|---|---|
| Pressure | cm $H_2O$ | kilopascal (kPa) | 0.09806 |
| | mm Hg (torr) | kPa | 0.1333 |
| | lb/in$^2$ (psi) | kPa | 6.895 |
| Compliance | L/cm $H_2O$ | L/k/Pa | 10.20 |
| Resistance | cm $H_2O$/L/sec | kPa/L/sec | 0.09806 |
| Work | kilogram-meter (kg-M) | joule (J) | 9.807 |
| Length | inch (in.) | meter (m) | 0.0254 |
| | foot (ft) | m | 0.3048 |
| Area | in.$^2$ | cm$^2$ | 6.452 |
| Volume | ft$^3$ | liter (L) | 28.32 |

**EXAMPLES**

To convert a conventional unit to an SI unit, *multiply* the conventional unit by the conversion factor. For example, convert 40 mm Hg to kPa:

40 mm Hg = 40 × 0.1333 = 5.33 kPa.

To convert an SI unit to a conventional unit, *divide* the SI unit by the conversion factor. For example, convert 350 kPa to lb/in$^2$ (psi):

$$350 \text{ kPa} = \frac{350}{6.895} = 50.76 \text{ psi.}$$

**REFERENCE**

Pierson

# Conversions of Other Units of Measurement

The following tables are from Des Jardins, T.R., *Cardiopulmonary Anatomy and Physiology: Essentials for Respiratory Care*, 3rd ed., Albany, NY: Delmar Publishers Inc., 1998. Used with permission.

## Metric Weight

| GRAMS | CENTIGRAMS | MILLIGRAMS | MICROGRAMS | NANOGRAMS |
|---|---|---|---|---|
| 1 | 100 | 1000 | 1,000,000 | 1,000,000,000 |
| 0.01 | 1 | 10 | 10,000 | 10,000,000 |
| 0.001 | 0.1 | 1 | 1000 | 1,000,000 |
| 0.000001 | 0.0001 | 0.001 | 1 | 1000 |
| 0.000000001 | 0.0000001 | 0.000001 | 0.001 | 1 |

## Metric Liquid

| LITER | CENTILITER | MILLILITER | MICROLITER | NANOLITER |
|---|---|---|---|---|
| 1 | 100 | 1000 | 1,000,000 | 1,000,000,000 |
| 0.01 | 1 | 10 | 10,000 | 10,000,000 |
| 0.001 | 0.1 | 1 | 1000 | 1,000,000 |
| 0.000001 | 0.0001 | 0.001 | 1 | 1000 |
| 0.000000001 | 0.0000001 | 0.000001 | 0.001 | 1 |

## Metric Length

| METER | CENTIMETER | MILLIMETER | MICROMETER | NANOMETER |
|---|---|---|---|---|
| 1 | 100 | 1000 | 1,000,000 | 1,000,000,000 |
| 0.01 | 1 | 10 | 10,000 | 10,000,000 |
| 0.001 | 0.1 | 1 | 1000 | 1,000,000 |
| 0.000001 | 0.0001 | 0.001 | 1 | 1000 |
| 0.000000001 | 0.0000001 | 0.000001 | 0.001 | 1 |

## Weight Conversions (Metric and Avoirdupois)

| GRAMS | KILOGRAMS | OUNCES | POUNDS |
|---|---|---|---|
| 1 | 0.001 | 0.0353 | 0.0022 |
| 1000 | 1 | 35.3 | 2.2 |
| 28.41 | 0.02841 | 1 | 1/16 |
| 454.5 | 0.4545 | 16 | 1 |

### Weight Conversions (Metric and Apothecary)

| GRAMS | MILLIGRAMS | GRAINS | DRAMS | OUNCES | POUNDS |
|---|---|---|---|---|---|
| 1 | 1000 | 15.4 | 0.2577 | 0.0322 | 0.00268 |
| 0.001 | 1 | 0.0154 | 0.00026 | 0.0000322 | 0.00000268 |
| 0.0648 | 64.8 | 1 | 1/60 | 1/480 | 1/5760 |
| 3.888 | 3888 | 60 | 1 | 1/8 | 1/96 |
| 31.1 | 31104 | 480 | 8 | 1 | 1/12 |
| 373.25 | 373248 | 5760 | 96 | 12 | 1 |

### Weight

| METRIC | APPROXIMATE APOTHECARY EQUIVALENTS |
|---|---|
| Grams | Grains |
| 0.0002 | 1/300 |
| 0.0003 | 1/200 |
| 0.0004 | 1/150 |
| 0.0005 | 1/120 |
| 0.0006 | 1/100 |
| 0.001 | 1/60 |
| 0.002 | 1/30 |
| 0.005 | 1/12 |
| 0.010 | 1/6 |
| 0.015 | 1/4 |
| 0.025 | 3/8 |
| 0.030 | 1/2 |
| 0.050 | 3/4 |
| 0.060 | 1 |
| 0.100 | 1 1/2 |
| 0.120 | 2 |
| 0.200 | 3 |
| 0.300 | 5 |
| 0.500 | 7 1/2 |
| 0.600 | 10 |
| 1 | 15 |
| 2 | 30 |
| 4 | 60 |

## Liquid Measure

| METRIC<br>*Milliliters* | APPROXIMATE APOTHECARY<br>EQUIVALENTS |
|---|---|
| 1000 | 1 quart |
| 750 | 1½ pints |
| 500 | 1 pint |
| 250 | 8 fluid ounces |
| 200 | 7 fluid ounces |
| 100 | 3½ fluid ounces |
| 50 | 1¾ fluid ounces |
| 30 | 1 fluid ounce |
| 15 | 4 fluid drams |
| 10 | 2½ fluid drams |
| 8 | 2 fluid drams |
| 5 | 1¼ fluid drams |
| 4 | 1 fluid dram |
| 3 | 45 minims |
| 2 | 30 minims |
| 1 | 15 minims |
| 0.75 | 12 minims |
| 0.6 | 10 minims |
| 0.5 | 8 minims |
| 0.3 | 5 minims |
| 0.25 | 4 minims |
| 0.2 | 3 minims |
| 0.1 | 1½ minims |
| 0.06 | 1 minim |
| 0.05 | ¾ minim |
| 0.03 | ½ minim |

## Volume Conversions: (Metric and Apothecary)

| MILLILITERS | MINIMS | FLUID<br>DRAMS | FLUID<br>OUNCES | PINTS | LITERS | GALLONS | QUARTS | FLUID<br>OUNCES | PINTS |
|---|---|---|---|---|---|---|---|---|---|
| 1 | 16.2 | 0.27 | 0.0338 | 0.0021 | 1 | 0.2642 | 1.057 | 33.824 | 2.114 |
| 0.0616 | 1 | 1/60 | 1/480 | 1/7680 | 3.785 | 1 | 4 | 128 | 8 |
| 3.697 | 60 | 1 | 1/8 | 1/128 | 0.946 | ¼ | 1 | 32 | 2 |
| 29.58 | 480 | 8 | 1 | 1/16 | 0.473 | 1/8 | ½ | 16 | 1 |
| 473.2 | 7680 | 128 | 16 | 1 | 0.0296 | 1/128 | 1/32 | 1 | 1/16 |

## Length Conversions (Metric and English System)

| | | MILLIMETERS | CENTIMETERS | INCHES | FEET | YARDS | METERS |
|---|---|---|---|---|---|---|---|
| 1 Å | = | $\dfrac{1}{10,000,000}$ | $\dfrac{1}{100,000,000}$ | $\dfrac{1}{254,000,000}$ | $\dfrac{1}{3,050,000,000}$ | $\dfrac{1}{9,140,000,000}$ | $\dfrac{1}{10,000,000,000}$ |
| 1 nm | = | $\dfrac{1}{1,000,000}$ | $\dfrac{1}{10,000,000}$ | $\dfrac{1}{25,400,000}$ | $\dfrac{1}{305,000,000}$ | $\dfrac{1}{914,000,000}$ | $\dfrac{1}{1,000,000,000}$ |
| 1 μ | = | $\dfrac{1}{1000}$ | $\dfrac{1}{10,000}$ | $\dfrac{1}{25,400}$ | $\dfrac{1}{305,000}$ | $\dfrac{1}{914,000}$ | $\dfrac{1}{1,000,000}$ |
| 1 mm | = | 1.0 | 0.1 | 0.03937 | 0.00328 | 0.0011 | 0.001 |
| 1 cm | = | 10.0 | 1.0 | 0.3937 | 0.03281 | 0.0109 | 0.01 |
| 1 in. | = | 25.4 | 2.54 | 1.0 | 0.0833 | 0.0278 | 0.0254 |
| 1 ft | = | 304.8 | 30.48 | 12.0 | 1.0 | 0.333 | 0.3048 |
| 1 yd | = | 914.40 | 91.44 | 36.0 | 3.0 | 1.0 | 0.9144 |
| 1 m | = | 1000.0 | 100.0 | 39.37 | 3.2808 | 1.0936 | 1.0 |

# Appendices

## Appendix A Partial Pressure (in mm Hg) of Gases in the air, Alveoli, and Blood*

| GASES | DRY AIR | ALVEOLAR GAS | ARTERIAL BLOOD | VENOUS BLOOD |
|---|---|---|---|---|
| $PO_2$ | 159.0 | 100.0 | 95.0 | 40.0 |
| $PO_2$ | 0.2 | 40.0 | 40.0 | 46.0 |
| $PH_2O$ (water vapor) | 0.0 | 47.0 | 47.0 | 47.0 |
| $PN_2$ (and other gases in minute quantities) | 600.8 | 573.0 | 573.0 | 573.0 |
| Total | 760.0 | 760.0 | 755.0 | 706.0 |

*The values shown are based upon standard pressure and temperature.
From Des Jardins, T.R. *Cardiopulmonary Anatomy and Physiology: Essentials for Respiratory Care,* 3rd ed. Albany, NY: Delmar Publishers, 1998.

## Appendix B $P_AO_2$ at Selected $F_IO_2$

| $F_IO_2$* | CALCULATED $P_AO_2$** |
|---|---|
| 21% | 100 |
| 25% | 128 |
| 30% | 164 |
| 35% | 200 |
| 40% | 235 |
| 45% | 271 |
| 50% | 307 |
| 55% | 342 |
| 60% | 388 |
| 65% | 423 |
| 70% | 459 |
| 75% | 495 |
| 80% | 530 |
| 85% | 566 |
| 90% | 602 |
| 95% | 637 |
| 100% | 673 |

*At $F_IO_2$ of 60% or higher, the factor 1.25 in the equation is omitted.
**The calculated $P_AO_2$ is based on a $PCO_2$ of 40 mm Hg, saturated at 37 °C, $P_B$ of 760 mm Hg. $P_AO_2 = (P_B - 47) \times F_IO_2 - (PCO_2 \times 1.25)$.
SEE: Alveolar Oxygen Tension ($P_AO_2$).

# Appendix C  Normal Electrolyte Concentrations in Plasma

| CATIONS | CONCENTRATION (RANGE) mEq/L | ANIONS | CONCENTRATION (RANGE) mEq/L |
|---|---|---|---|
| $Na^+$ | 140 (138 to 142) | $Cl^-$ | 103 (101 to 105) |
| $K^+$ | 4 (3 to 5) | $HCO_3^-$ | 25 (23 to 27) |
| $Ca^{++}$ | 5 (4.5 to 5.5) | Protein | 16 (14 to 18) |
| $Mg^{++}$ | 2 (1.5 to 2.5) | $HPO_4^{--}$, $H_2PO_4^-$ | 2 (1.5 to 2.5) |
| Total | 151 | $SO_4^{--}$ | 1 (0.8 to 1.2) |
| | | Organic acids | 4 (3.5 to 4.5) |
| | | Total | 151 |

# Appendix D  Oxygen Transport Normal Ranges

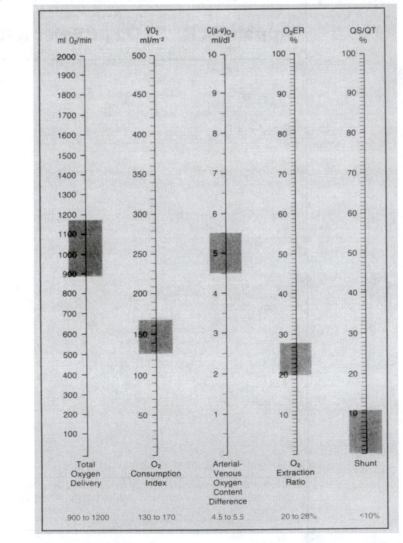

| Total Oxygen Delivery | $O_2$ Consumption Index | Arterial-Venous Oxygen Content Difference | $O_2$ Extraction Ratio | Shunt |
|---|---|---|---|---|
| 900 to 1200 | 130 to 170 | 4.5 to 5.5 | 20 to 28% | <10% |

From Des Jardins, T.R. *Cardiopulmonary Anatomy and Physiology: Essentials for Respiratory Care*, 3rd ed. Albany, NY: Delmar Publishers, 1998.

# Appendix E Factors for Converting Gas Volumes from ATPS to BTPS

| GAS TEMPERATURE (°C) | FACTORS TO CONVERT TO 37°C SATURATED* | WATER VAPOR PRESSURE (mm Hg) |
|---|---|---|
| 18 | 1.112 | 15.6 |
| 19 | 1.107 | 16.5 |
| 20 | 1.102 | 17.5 |
| 21 | 1.096 | 18.7 |
| 22 | 1.091 | 19.8 |
| 23 | 1.085 | 21.1 |
| 24 | 1.080 | 22.4 |
| 25 | 1.075 | 23.8 |
| 26 | 1.068 | 25.2 |
| 27 | 1.063 | 26.7 |
| 28 | 1.057 | 28.3 |
| 29 | 1.051 | 30.0 |
| 30 | 1.045 | 31.8 |
| 31 | 1.039 | 33.7 |
| 32 | 1.032 | 35.7 |
| 33 | 1.026 | 37.7 |
| 34 | 1.020 | 39.9 |
| 35 | 1.014 | 42.2 |
| 36 | 1.007 | 44.6 |
| 37 | 1.000 | 47.0 |
| 38 | 0.993 | 49.8 |
| 39 | 0.986 | 52.5 |
| 40 | 0.979 | 55.4 |
| 41 | 0.971 | 58.4 |
| 42 | 0.964 | 61.6 |

*Conversion factors are based on $P_B = 760$ mm Hg. For other barometric pressures and temperatures, use the following equation: Conversion factor $= \dfrac{P_B - PH_2O}{P_B - 47} \times \dfrac{310}{(273 + °C)}$

# Appendix F  DuBois Body Surface Chart

## Directions

To find body surface of a patient, locate the height in inches (or centimeters) on Scale I and the weight in pounds (or kilograms) on Scale II and place a straight edge (ruler) between these two points, which will intersect Scale III at the patient's surface area.

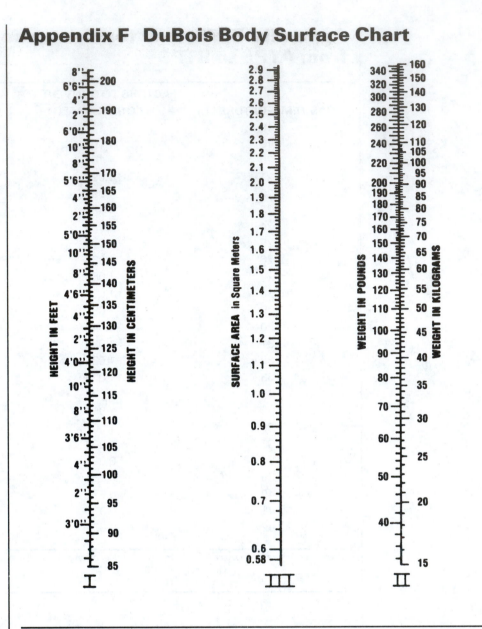

Adapted from DuBois, Eugene F. *Basal Metabolism in Health and Disease*. Philadelphia: Lea and Febiger, 1924.

# Appendix G  Hemodynamic Normal Ranges

**Hemodynamic Values Directly Obtained by Means of the Pulmonary Artery Catheter**

| HEMODYNAMIC VALUE | ABBREVIATION | NORMAL RANGE |
|---|---|---|
| Central venous pressure | CVP | 1 to 7 mm Hg |
| Right atrial pressure | RAP | 1 to 7 mm Hg |
| Mean pulmonary artery pressure | $\overline{PA}$ | 15 mm Hg |
| Pulmonary capillary wedge pressure | PCWP | 8 to 12 mm Hg |
| (also called pulmonary artery | PAW | |
| wedge; pulmonary artery occlusion) | PAO | |
| Cardiac output | CO | 4 to 8 L/min |

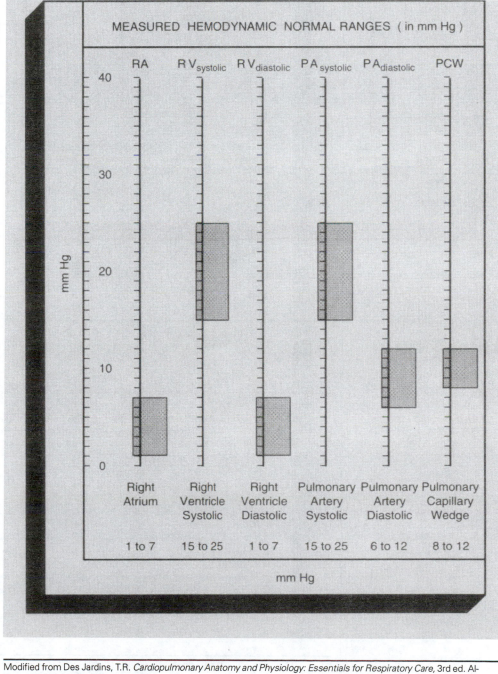

Modified from Des Jardins, T.R. *Cardiopulmonary Anatomy and Physiology: Essentials for Respiratory Care*, 3rd ed. Albany, NY: Delmar Publishers, 1998.

## Computed Hemodynamic Values

| HEMODYNAMIC VARIABLE | ABBREVIATION | NORMAL RANGE |
|---|:---:|:---:|
| Stroke volume | SV | 40 to 80 mL |
| Stroke volume index | SVI | 33 to 47 L/beat/m$^2$ |
| Cardiac index | CI | 2.5 to 3.5 L/min/m$^2$ |
| Right ventricular stroke work index | RVSWI | 7 to 12 g · m/beat/m$^2$ |
| Left ventricular stroke work index | LVSWI | 40 to 60 g · m/beat/m$^2$ |
| Pulmonary vascular resistance | PVR | 50 to 150 dyne·sec/cm$^5$ |
| Systemic vascular resistance | SVR | 800 to 1500 dyne·sec/cm$^5$ |

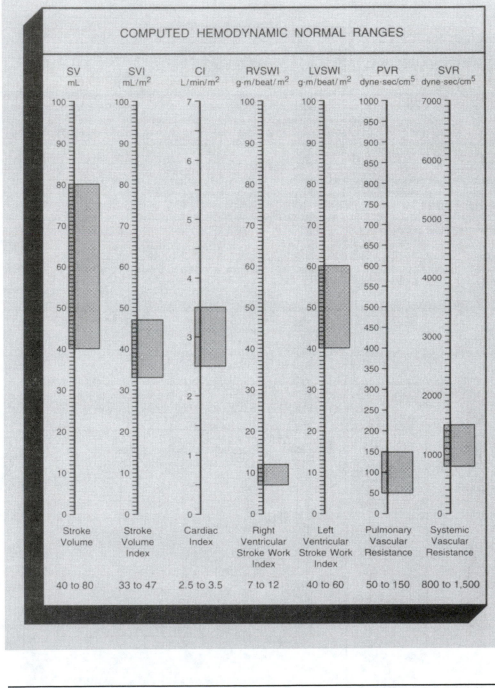

Modified from Des Jardins, T.R. *Cardiopulmonary Anatomy and Physiology: Essentials for Respiratory Care,* 3rd ed. Albany, NY: Delmar Publishers, 1998.

# Appendix H   Periodic Chart of Elements

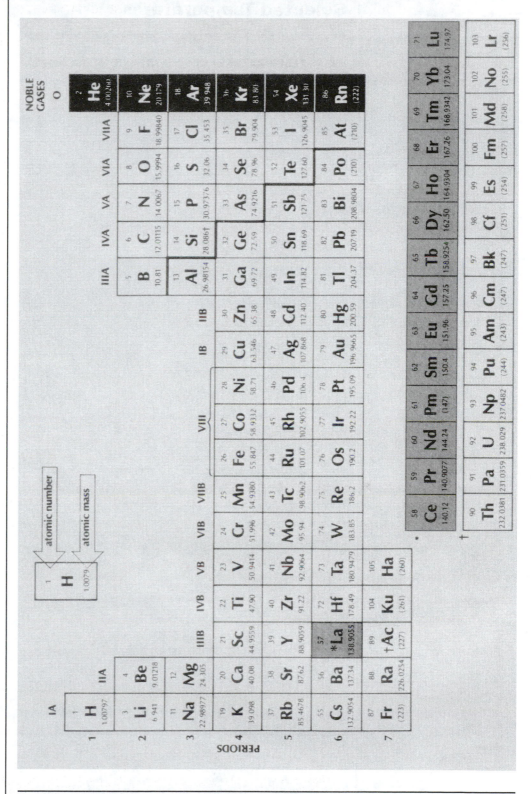

From Malone, Leo J.; *Basic Concepts of Chemistry,* 5th ed. © 1981. Reprinted by permission of John Wiley & Sons, Inc.

# Appendix I  Humidity Capacity of Saturated Gas at Selected Temperatures

| GAS TEMPERATURE (°C) | WATER CONTENT (mg/L) | WATER VAPOR PRESSURE (mm Hg) |
|---|---|---|
| 0 | 4.9 | 4.6 |
| 5 | 6.8 | 6.6 |
| 10 | 9.4 | 9.3 |
| 17 | 14.5 | 14.6 |
| 18 | 15.4 | 15.6 |
| 19 | 16.3 | 16.5 |
| 20 | 17.3 | 17.5 |
| 21 | 18.4 | 18.7 |
| 22 | 19.4 | 19.8 |
| 23 | 20.6 | 21.1 |
| 24 | 21.8 | 22.4 |
| 25 | 23.1 | 23.8 |
| 26 | 24.4 | 25.2 |
| 27 | 25.8 | 26.7 |
| 28 | 27.2 | 28.3 |
| 29 | 28.8 | 30.0 |
| 30 | 30.4 | 31.8 |
| 31 | 32.0 | 33.7 |
| 32 | 33.8 | 35.7 |
| 33 | 35.6 | 37.7 |
| 34 | 37.6 | 39.9 |
| 35 | 39.6 | 42.2 |
| 36 | 41.7 | 44.6 |
| 37 | 43.9 | 47.0 |
| 38 | 46.2 | 49.8 |
| 39 | 48.6 | 52.5 |
| 40 | 51.1 | 55.4 |
| 41 | 53.7 | 58.4 |
| 42 | 56.5 | 61.6 |
| 43 | 59.5 | 64.9 |

# Appendix J  Normal Values for Lung Volumes, Capacities, and Ventilation

| VOLUME | NEWBORN INFANT | YOUNG ADULT MALE | APPROX. % OF TLC (YOUNG ADULT MALE) |
|---|---|---|---|
| $V_T$ (mL) | 15 | 500 | 8 to 10 |
| $IRV$ (mL) | 60 | 3100 | 50 |
| $ERV$ (mL) | 40 | 1200 | 20 |
| $RV$ (mL) | 40 | 1200 | 20 |
| $IC$ (mL) | 75 | 3600 | 60 |
| $FRC$ (mL) | 80 | 2400 | 40 |
| $VC$ (mL) | 115 | 4800 | 80 |
| $TLC$ (mL) | 155 | 6000 | 100 |
| $f$ (bpm) | 35 to 50 | 12 to 20 | |
| $\dot{V}_E$ | 525 to 750 mL/min | 6 to 10 L/min | |

Modified from Madama, V.C. *Pulmonary Function Testing and Cardiopulmonary Stress Testing*, 2nd ed. Albany, NY: Delmar Publishers, 1998.

# Appendix K  Conversion Factors for Calculating Duration of Gas Cylinders

| CYLINDER SIZE | B/BB | D/DD | E | M | G | H/K |
|---|---|---|---|---|---|---|
| Carbon Dioxide ($CO_2$) | 0.17 | 0.43 | 0.72 | 3.44 | 5.59 | 7.18 |
| Carbon Dioxide/Oxygen ($CO_2/O_2$) | | 0.18 | 0.3 | 1.36 | 2.42 | 2.73 |
| Cyclopropane ($C_3H_6$) | 0.17 | 0.40 | | | | |
| Helium (He) | | 0.14 | 0.23 | 1.03 | 1.82 | 2.73 |
| Helium/Oxygen ($He/O_2$) | | | 0.23 | 1.03 | 1.82 | 2.05 |
| Nitrous Oxide ($N_2O$) | | 0.43 | 0.72 | 3.44 | 6.27 | 7.18 |
| Oxygen ($O_2$) | 0.09 | 0.18 | 0.28 | 1.57 | 2.41 | 3.14 |
| Air ($N_2/O_2$) | | 0.17 | 0.28 | 1.49 | 2.30 | 2.98 |
| Nitrogen ($N_2$) | | | 0.28 | | | 2.91 |

*(Conversion factors are based on full cylinder at pressure of 2200 psig.)*
*To calculate duration of gas cylinder at a constant liter flow: (1) multiply the conversion factor by the pressure reading on the gas gauge; (2) divide the product from (1) by the liter flow in use; (3) answer equals the duration, in minutes, of gas cylinder at the same liter flow.*

$$Duration = \frac{Conversion\ factor \times psig}{Liter\ flow}$$

*For example, see Oxygen Duration of E Cylinder and Oxygen Duration of H or K Cylinder.*

# REFERENCE  White

## Appendix L Barometric Pressures at Selected Altitudes

| | FEET | METERS | $P_B$ (mm Hg) |
|---|---|---|---|
| Below sea | −66 | −20 | 2,280 |
| level | −33 | −10 | 1,520 |
| Sea level | 0 | 0 | 760 |
| Above sea level | 2,000 | 610 | 707 |
| | 4,000 | 1,219 | 656 |
| | 6,000[a] | 1,829 | 609 |
| | 8,000 | 2,438 | 564 |
| | 10,000 | 3,048 | 523 |
| | 12,000 | 3,658 | 483 |
| | 14,000[b] | 4,267 | 446 |
| | 16,000 | 4,877 | 412 |
| | 18,000 | 5,486 | 379 |
| | 20,000 | 6,096 | 349 |
| | 22,000 | 6,706 | 321 |
| | 24,000 | 7,315 | 294 |
| | 26,000 | 7,925 | 270 |
| | 28,000 | 8,534 | 247 |
| | 30,000[c] | 9,144 | 226 |
| | 32,000 | 9,754 | 206 |
| | 34,000 | 10,363 | 187 |
| | 36,000 | 10,973 | 170 |
| | 40,000 | 12,192 | 141 |
| | 50,000 | 15,240 | 87 |
| | 63,000 | 19,202 | 47 |

[a] Denver, Colorado, 5,280 ft
[b] Mount Elbert, Colorado, 14,433 ft
[c] Mount Everest, 29,028 ft

## Appendix M   Using the Logarithm Table

**TERMI-NOLOGY**

$\log 20 = 1.301$
↓ ↓ ↓ ↓
a  b  c  d

a: logarithm, b: number, c: characteristic, d: mantissa.

**EXAMPLE 1**

Find the logarithm for 30.4.

Step 1. From the log table find the number 30 along the vertical column (N).

Step 2. Find the number 4 along the horizontal row (N).

Step 3. The mantissa intersected by the column and row should read 4829.

Step 4. Since the number 30.4 has two digits in front of the decimal point, use 1. in front of the mantissa. Log 30.4 becomes 1.4829.

**NOTE**

The characteristic is determined by the number of digits in front of the decimal point. The characteristic is 0. for one digit in front of the decimal point; 1. for two digits; 2. for three digits; and so on.

For example, the answer for log 304 is 2.4829. You may notice that the mantissa for 304 is same as that for 30.4 and that the only change is in the characteristic. The following examples should clarify this point:

log 0.0304 = $\overline{2}$.4829

log 0.304 = $\overline{1}$.4829

log 3.04 = 0.4829

log 30.4 = 1.4829

log 304 = 2.4829

log 3040 = 3.4829

**EXAMPLE 2**

Find the logarithms for 18.7 and 187.

Step 1. From the log table find the number 18 along the vertical column (N).

Step 2. Find the number 7 along the horizontal row (N).

Step 3. The mantissa intersected by the column and row should read 2718.

Step 4. Since the number 18.7 has two digits in front of the decimal point, use 1. in front of the mantissa. Log 18.7 becomes 1.2718. Since the number 187 has three digits in front of the decimal point, use 2. in front of the mantissa. Log 187 becomes 2.2718.

**EXERCISE 1**

Find the logarithm for 22.2.

[Answer: log 22.2 = 1.3464]

**EXERCISE 2**

Find the logarithm for 30.15.

[Answer: log 30.15 = 1.4793. Look for the mantissas under 1 and 2 and find the average.]

## Common Logarithms of Numbers[a]

| N | 0 | 1 | 2 | 3 | 4 | 5 | 6 | 7 | 8 | 9 |
|----|------|------|------|------|------|------|------|------|------|------|
| 10 | 0000 | 0043 | 0086 | 0128 | 0170 | 0212 | 0253 | 0294 | 0334 | 0374 |
| 11 | 0414 | 0453 | 0492 | 0531 | 0569 | 0607 | 0645 | 0682 | 0719 | 0755 |
| 12 | 0792 | 0828 | 0864 | 0899 | 0934 | 0969 | 1004 | 1038 | 1072 | 1106 |
| 13 | 1139 | 1173 | 1206 | 1239 | 1271 | 1303 | 1335 | 1367 | 1399 | 1430 |
| 14 | 1461 | 1492 | 1523 | 1553 | 1584 | 1614 | 1644 | 1673 | 1703 | 1732 |
| 15 | 1761 | 1790 | 1818 | 1847 | 1875 | 1903 | 1931 | 1959 | 1987 | 2014 |
| 16 | 2041 | 2068 | 2095 | 2122 | 2148 | 2175 | 2201 | 2227 | 2253 | 2279 |
| 17 | 2304 | 2330 | 2335 | 2380 | 2405 | 2430 | 2455 | 2480 | 2504 | 2529 |
| 18 | 2553 | 2577 | 2601 | 2625 | 2648 | 2672 | 2695 | 2718 | 2742 | 2765 |
| 19 | 2788 | 2810 | 2833 | 2856 | 2878 | 2900 | 2923 | 2945 | 2967 | 2989 |
| 20 | 3010 | 3032 | 3054 | 3075 | 3096 | 3118 | 3139 | 3160 | 3181 | 3201 |
| 21 | 3222 | 3243 | 3263 | 3284 | 3304 | 3324 | 3345 | 3365 | 3385 | 3404 |
| 22 | 3424 | 3444 | 3464 | 3483 | 3502 | 3522 | 3541 | 3560 | 3579 | 3598 |
| 23 | 3617 | 3636 | 3655 | 3674 | 3692 | 3711 | 3729 | 3747 | 3766 | 3784 |
| 24 | 3802 | 3820 | 3838 | 3856 | 3874 | 3892 | 3909 | 3927 | 3945 | 3962 |
| 25 | 3979 | 3997 | 4014 | 4031 | 4048 | 4065 | 4082 | 4099 | 4116 | 4133 |
| 26 | 4150 | 4166 | 4183 | 4200 | 4216 | 4232 | 4249 | 4265 | 4281 | 4298 |
| 27 | 4314 | 4330 | 4346 | 4362 | 4378 | 4393 | 4409 | 4425 | 4440 | 4456 |
| 28 | 4472 | 4487 | 4502 | 4518 | 4533 | 4548 | 4564 | 4579 | 4594 | 4609 |
| 29 | 4624 | 4639 | 4654 | 4669 | 4683 | 4698 | 4713 | 4728 | 4742 | 4757 |
| 30 | 4771 | 4786 | 4800 | 4814 | 4829 | 4843 | 4857 | 4871 | 4886 | 4900 |
| 31 | 4914 | 4928 | 4942 | 4955 | 4969 | 4983 | 4997 | 5011 | 5024 | 5038 |
| 32 | 5051 | 5065 | 5079 | 5092 | 5105 | 5119 | 5132 | 5145 | 5159 | 5172 |
| 33 | 5185 | 5198 | 5211 | 5224 | 5237 | 5250 | 5263 | 5276 | 5289 | 5302 |
| 34 | 5315 | 5328 | 5340 | 5353 | 5366 | 5378 | 5391 | 5403 | 5416 | 5428 |
| 35 | 5441 | 5453 | 5465 | 5478 | 5490 | 5502 | 5514 | 5527 | 5539 | 5551 |
| 36 | 5563 | 5575 | 5587 | 5599 | 5611 | 5623 | 5635 | 5647 | 5658 | 5670 |
| 37 | 5682 | 5694 | 5705 | 5717 | 5729 | 5740 | 5752 | 5763 | 5775 | 5786 |
| 38 | 5798 | 5809 | 5821 | 5832 | 5843 | 5855 | 5866 | 5877 | 5888 | 5899 |
| 39 | 5911 | 5922 | 5933 | 5944 | 5955 | 5966 | 5977 | 5988 | 5999 | 6010 |
| 40 | 6021 | 6031 | 6042 | 6053 | 6064 | 6075 | 6085 | 6096 | 6107 | 6117 |
| 41 | 6128 | 6138 | 6149 | 6160 | 6170 | 6180 | 6191 | 6201 | 6212 | 6222 |
| 42 | 6232 | 6243 | 6253 | 6263 | 6274 | 6284 | 6294 | 6304 | 6314 | 6325 |
| 43 | 6335 | 6345 | 6355 | 6365 | 6375 | 6385 | 6395 | 6405 | 6415 | 6425 |
| 44 | 6435 | 6444 | 6454 | 6464 | 6474 | 6484 | 6493 | 6503 | 6513 | 6522 |
| 45 | 6532 | 6542 | 6551 | 6561 | 6571 | 6580 | 6590 | 6599 | 6609 | 6618 |
| 46 | 6628 | 6637 | 6646 | 6656 | 6665 | 6675 | 6684 | 6693 | 6702 | 6712 |
| 47 | 6721 | 6730 | 6739 | 6749 | 6758 | 6767 | 6776 | 6785 | 6794 | 6803 |
| 48 | 6812 | 6821 | 6830 | 6839 | 6848 | 6857 | 6866 | 6875 | 6884 | 6893 |
| 49 | 6902 | 6911 | 6920 | 6928 | 6937 | 6946 | 6955 | 6964 | 6972 | 6981 |
| 50 | 6990 | 6998 | 7007 | 7016 | 7024 | 7033 | 7042 | 7050 | 7059 | 7067 |
| 51 | 7076 | 7084 | 7093 | 7101 | 7110 | 7118 | 7126 | 7135 | 7143 | 7152 |
| 52 | 7160 | 7168 | 7177 | 7185 | 7193 | 7202 | 7210 | 7218 | 7226 | 7235 |
| 53 | 7243 | 7251 | 7259 | 7267 | 7275 | 7284 | 7292 | 7300 | 7308 | 7316 |
| 54 | 7324 | 7332 | 7340 | 7348 | 7356 | 7364 | 7372 | 7380 | 7388 | 7396 |
| 55 | 7404 | 7412 | 7419 | 7427 | 7435 | 7443 | 7451 | 7459 | 7466 | 7474 |
| 56 | 7482 | 7490 | 7497 | 7505 | 7513 | 7520 | 7528 | 7536 | 7543 | 7551 |
| 57 | 7559 | 7566 | 7574 | 7582 | 7589 | 7597 | 7604 | 7612 | 7619 | 7627 |

| N | 0 | 1 | 2 | 3 | 4 | 5 | 6 | 7 | 8 | 9 |
|---|---|---|---|---|---|---|---|---|---|---|
| 58 | 7634 | 7642 | 7649 | 7657 | 7664 | 7672 | 7679 | 7686 | 7694 | 7701 |
| 59 | 7709 | 7716 | 7723 | 7731 | 7738 | 7745 | 7752 | 7760 | 7767 | 7774 |
| 60 | 7782 | 7789 | 7796 | 7803 | 7810 | 7818 | 7825 | 7832 | 7839 | 7846 |
| 61 | 7853 | 7860 | 7868 | 7875 | 7892 | 7889 | 7896 | 7903 | 7910 | 7917 |
| 62 | 7924 | 7931 | 7938 | 7945 | 7952 | 7959 | 7966 | 7973 | 7980 | 7987 |
| 63 | 7993 | 8000 | 8007 | 8014 | 8021 | 8028 | 8035 | 8041 | 8048 | 8055 |
| 64 | 8062 | 8069 | 8075 | 8082 | 8089 | 8096 | 8102 | 8109 | 8116 | 8122 |
| 65 | 8129 | 8136 | 8142 | 8149 | 8156 | 8162 | 8169 | 8176 | 8182 | 8189 |
| 66 | 8195 | 8202 | 8209 | 8215 | 8222 | 8228 | 8235 | 8241 | 8248 | 8254 |
| 67 | 8261 | 8267 | 8274 | 8280 | 8287 | 8293 | 8299 | 8306 | 8312 | 8319 |
| 68 | 8325 | 8331 | 8338 | 8344 | 8351 | 8357 | 8363 | 8370 | 8376 | 8382 |
| 69 | 8388 | 8395 | 8401 | 8407 | 8414 | 8420 | 8426 | 8432 | 8439 | 8445 |
| 70 | 8451 | 8457 | 8463 | 8470 | 8476 | 8482 | 8488 | 8494 | 8500 | 8506 |
| 71 | 8513 | 8519 | 8525 | 8531 | 8537 | 8543 | 8549 | 8555 | 8561 | 8567 |
| 72 | 8573 | 8579 | 8585 | 8591 | 8597 | 8603 | 8609 | 8615 | 8621 | 8627 |
| 73 | 8633 | 8639 | 8645 | 8651 | 8657 | 8663 | 8669 | 8675 | 8681 | 8686 |
| 74 | 8692 | 8698 | 8704 | 8710 | 8716 | 8722 | 8727 | 8733 | 8739 | 8745 |
| 75 | 8751 | 8756 | 8762 | 8768 | 8774 | 8779 | 8785 | 8791 | 8797 | 8802 |
| 76 | 8808 | 8814 | 8820 | 8825 | 8831 | 8837 | 3342 | 8848 | 8854 | 8859 |
| 77 | 8865 | 8871 | 8876 | 8882 | 8887 | 8893 | 8899 | 8904 | 8910 | 8915 |
| 78 | 8921 | 8927 | 8932 | 8938 | 8943 | 8949 | 8954 | 8960 | 8965 | 8971 |
| 79 | 8976 | 8982 | 8987 | 8993 | 8998 | 9004 | 9009 | 9015 | 9020 | 9025 |
| 80 | 9031 | 9036 | 9042 | 9047 | 9053 | 9058 | 9063 | 9069 | 9074 | 9079 |
| 81 | 9085 | 9090 | 9096 | 9101 | 9106 | 9112 | 9117 | 9122 | 9128 | 9133 |
| 82 | 9138 | 9143 | 9149 | 9154 | 9159 | 9165 | 9170 | 9175 | 9180 | 9186 |
| 83 | 9191 | 9196 | 9201 | 9206 | 9212 | 9217 | 9222 | 9227 | 9232 | 9238 |
| 84 | 9243 | 9248 | 9253 | 9258 | 9263 | 9269 | 9274 | 9279 | 9284 | 9289 |
| 85 | 9294 | 9299 | 9304 | 9309 | 9315 | 9320 | 9325 | 9330 | 9335 | 9340 |
| 86 | 9345 | 9350 | 9355 | 9360 | 9365 | 9370 | 9375 | 9380 | 9385 | 9390 |
| 87 | 9395 | 9400 | 9405 | 9410 | 9415 | 9420 | 9425 | 9430 | 9435 | 9440 |
| 88 | 9445 | 9450 | 9455 | 9460 | 9465 | 9469 | 9474 | 9479 | 9484 | 9489 |
| 89 | 9494 | 9499 | 9504 | 9509 | 9513 | 9518 | 9523 | 9528 | 9533 | 9538 |
| 90 | 9542 | 9547 | 9552 | 9557 | 9562 | 9566 | 9571 | 9576 | 9581 | 9586 |
| 91 | 9590 | 9595 | 9600 | 9605 | 9609 | 9614 | 9619 | 9624 | 9628 | 9633 |
| 92 | 9638 | 9643 | 9647 | 9652 | 9657 | 9661 | 9666 | 9671 | 9675 | 9680 |
| 93 | 9685 | 9689 | 9694 | 9699 | 9703 | 9708 | 9713 | 9714 | 9722 | 9727 |
| 94 | 9731 | 9736 | 9741 | 9745 | 9750 | 9754 | 9759 | 9763 | 9768 | 9773 |
| 95 | 9777 | 9782 | 9786 | 9791 | 9795 | 9800 | 9805 | 9809 | 9814 | 9818 |
| 96 | 9823 | 9827 | 9832 | 9836 | 9841 | 9845 | 9850 | 9854 | 9859 | 9863 |
| 97 | 9868 | 9872 | 9877 | 9881 | 9886 | 9890 | 9894 | 9899 | 9903 | 9908 |
| 98 | 9912 | 9917 | 9921 | 9926 | 9930 | 9934 | 9939 | 9943 | 9948 | 9952 |
| 99 | 9956 | 9961 | 9965 | 9969 | 9974 | 9978 | 9983 | 9987 | 9991 | 9996 |

[a] This table gives the mantissas of numbers with the decimal point omitted in each case. Characteristics are determined by inspection from the numbers.
From Wojciechowski, W.V. *Respiratory Care Sciences: An Integrated Approach*, 2nd ed. Albany, NY: Delmar Publishers, 1996.

# Bibliography

Barnes, T.A., et al. *Core Textbook of Respiratory Care Practice.* St. Louis: Mosby Year-Book, 1993.

Burton, G.G., et al. *Respiratory Care: A Guide to Clinical Practice.* 3rd ed. Philadelphia: J.B. Lippincott, 1991.

Bustin, D. *Hemodynamic Monitoring for Critical Care.* Norwalk, Connecticut: Appleton-Century-Crofts, 1986.

Chatburn, R.L., et al. *Fundamentals of Respiratory Care Research.* East Norwalk, Connecticut: Appleton & Lange, 1988.

Des Jardins, T.R. *Cardiopulmonary Anatomy and Physiology: Essentials for Respiratory Care.* 3rd ed. Albany, New York: Delmar Publishers, 1998.

Dupuis, Y.G. *Ventilators: Theory and Clinical Application.* St. Louis: C.V. Mosby, 1986.

Grauer, K., et al. *ACLS Certification Preparation and a Comprehensive Review.* 3rd ed. St. Louis: C.V. Mosby, 1993.

Gross, L.J. "Setting Cutoff Scores on Credentialing Examinations: A refinement in the Nedelsky Procedure." *Evaluation and the Health Professions* 8:4, 469–493 (1985).

Hegstad, L.N., et al. *Essential Drug Dosage Calcuations.* Maryland: Robert J. Brady, 1983.

Jabour, E.R., et al. "Evaluation of a new weaning index based on ventilatory endurance and the efficiency of gas exchange." *Am Rev Respir Dis* 144:531-537 (1991).

Kacmarek, R.M., et al. *The Essentials of Respiratory Therapy.* 2nd ed. Chicago: Year-Book Medical Publishers, 1985.

Koff, P.B., et al. *Neonatal and Pediatric Respiratory Care.* St. Louis: C.V. Mosby, 1988.

Krider, T.M., et al., *Master Guide for Passing the Respiratory Care Credentialing Exams.* Claremont, California: Education Resource Consortium, 1986.

Madama, V.C. *Pulmonary Function Testing and Cardiopulmonary Stress Testing.* 2nd ed. Albany, New York: Delmar Publishers, 1998.

Malasanos, L., et al. *Health Assessment.* 2nd ed. St. Louis: C.V. Mosby, 1981.

Malley, W.J. *Clinical Blood Gases: Application and Noninvasive Alternatives.* Philadelphia: W.B. Saunders, 1990.

McIntyre, K.M., et al. *Textbook of Advanced Cardiac Life Support.* Dallas: American Heart Association, 1987.

McPherson, S.P. *Respiratory Home Care Equipment.* Dubuque, Iowa: Kendall/Hunt, 1988.

Moser, K.M., et al. *Respiratory Emergency.* St. Louis: C.V. Mosby, 1982.

Nedelsky, L. "Absolute Grading Standards for Objective Tests." *Educational and Psychologic Measurement* 14: 3–19 (1954).

Pierson, D.J., et al. *Foundations of Respiratory Care.* New York: Churchill Livingstone, 1992.

Rattenborg, C.C. *Clinical Use of Mechanical Ventilation.* Chicago: Year-Book Medical Publishers, 1981.

Rau, J.L., Jr. *Respiratory Care Pharmacology.* 4th ed. St. Louis: Mosby Year-Book, 1993.

Ruppel, G.L. *Manual of Pulmonary Function Testing.* 6th ed. St. Louis: Mosby Year-Book, 1993.

Scanlan, C.L., et al. *Egan's Fundamentals of Respiratory Care.* 5th ed. St. Louis: C.V. Mosby, 1990.

Shapiro, B.A., et al. (1) *Clinical Application of Blood Gases.* 5th ed. St. Louis: Mosby Year-Book, 1993.

Shapiro, B.A., et al. (2) *Clinical Application of Respiratory Care.* 4th ed. St. Louis: Mosby Year-Book, 1990.

Tobin, M.J., et al. "The pattern of breathing during successful and unsuccessful trials of weaning from mechanical ventilation." *Am Rev Respir Dis* 134:1111-1118 (1986).

Tuckman, B.W. *Conducting Educational Research.* 2nd ed. New York: Harcourt Brace Jovanovich, 1978.

Whitaker, K.B., et al. *Comprehensive Perinatal and Pediatric Respiratory Care.* 2nd ed. Albany, New York: Delmar Publishers, 1998.

White, G.C. *Equipment Theory for Respiratory Care.* 2nd ed. Albany, New York: Delmar Publishers, 1996.

Wilkins, R.L., et al. *Clinical Assessment in Respiratory Care.* St. Louis: C.V. Mosby, 1985.

Wojciechowski, W.V. *Respiratory Care Sciences: An Integrated Approach.* 2nd ed. Albany, New York: Delmar Publishers, 1996.

Yang, K.L., et al. "A prospective study of indexes predicting the outcome of trials of weaning from mechanical ventilation." *N Engl J Med* 324:1445-1450 (1991).

# Index by Alphabetical Listing

Airway Resistance: Estimated ($R_{aw}$)   9

Alveolar–Arterial Oxygen Tension Gradient $P(A-a)O_2$   11

Alveolar Oxygen Tension ($P_AO_2$)   14

Anion Gap   16

Answer Key to Self-Assessment Questions   283

Arterial/Alveolar Oxygen Tension ($a/A$) Ratio   18

Arterial–Mixed Venous Oxygen Content Difference [$C(a-\bar{v})O_2$]   20

ATPS to BTPS   23


Barometric Pressures at Selected Altitudes (Appendix L)   316

Basic Statistics and Educational Calculations   261

Bibliography   321

Bicarbonate Corrections of Base Deficit   25

Body Surface Area   27


Cardiac Index ($CI$)   29

Cardiac Output ($CO$): Fick's Estimated Method   32

Common Logarithms of Numbers   318

Compliance: Dynamic ($C_{dyn}$)   35

Compliance: Static ($C_{st}$)   38

Compliance: Total ($C_T$)   41

Conversion Factors for Calculating Duration of Gas Cylinders (Appendix K)   315

Conversions of Conventional and Système International Units   300

Conversions of Other Units of Measurement   301

Corrected Tidal Volume ($V_T$)   43

Correction Factor   45

Cut Score: Revised Nedelsky Procedure   279


Dalton's Law of Partial Pressure   49

Deadspace to Tidal Volume Ratio ($V_D/V_T$)   51

Density ($D$) of Gases   54

Dosage Calculation: Intravenous Solution Infusion Dosage   57

Dosage Calculation: Intravenous Solution Infusion Rate   60

Dosage Calculation: Percent (%) Solutions   63

Dosage Calculation: Unit Dose   67

Dosage Estimation for Children: Young's Rule   72

Dosage Estimation for Infants and Children: Clark's Rule   74

Dosage Estimation for Infants and Children: Fried's Rule   76

DuBois Body Surface Chart (Appendix F)    310

Elastance ($E$)    78
Endotracheal Tube Size for Children    80

Factors for Converting Gas Volumes from ATPS to BTPS (Appendix E)    309
French (Fr) and Millimeter (mm) Conversions    299
Fick's Law of Diffusion    83
$F_IO_2$ from Two Gas Sources    86
$F_IO_2$ Needed for a Desired $P_aO_2$    89
$F_IO_2$ Needed for a Desired $P_aO_2$ (COPD Patients)    91
Flow Rate in Mechanical Ventilation    93
Forced Vital Capacity Tracing: $FEF_{200-1200}$    102
Forced Vital Capacity Tracing: $FEF_{25-75\%}$    110
Forced Vital Capacity Tracing: $FEV_t$ and $FEV_{t\%}$    95

Gas Law Equations    120
Gas Volume Corrections    123
Graham's Law of Diffusion Coefficient    126

Helium/Oxygen (He/$O_2$) Flow Rate Conversion    128
Hemodynamic Normal Ranges (Appendix G)    311
Humidity Capacity of Saturated Gas at Selected Temperatures (Appendix I)    314
Humidity Deficit    130

$I{:}E$ Ratio    132
Index by Alphabetical Listing    323

Kuder-Richardson Reliability Coefficient (K-R21)    275

Law of LaPlace    138
Listing by Subject Areas    vi
Lung Volumes and Capacities    140

Mean Airway Pressure ($MAWP$)    147
Mean Arterial Pressure ($MAP$)    151
Measures of Central Tendency    268
Metric Conversion–Length    153
Metric Conversion–Volume    156
Metric Conversion–Weight    159
Minute Ventilation during IMV    162
Minute Ventilation: Expired and Alveolar    164

Normal Electrolyte Concentrations in Plasma (Appendix C)    308
Normal Values for Lung Volumes, Capacities, and Ventilation (Appendix J)    315

Oxygen:Air ($O_2$:Air) Entrainment Ratio    168
Oxygen Consumption ($\dot{V}O_2$) and Index ($\dot{V}O_2$ Index)    172
Oxygen Content: Arterial ($C_aO_2$)    176

Oxygen Content: End-Capillary ($C_cO_2$)    180
Oxygen Content: Mixed Venous ($C_{\bar{v}}O_2$)    182
Oxygen Duration of E Cylinder    184
Oxygen Duration of H or K Cylinder    187
Oxygen Duration of Liquid System    190
Oxygen Extraction Ratio ($O_2ER$)    195
Oxygen Transport Normal Ranges (Appendix D)    308

$P_AO_2$ at Selected $F_IO_2$ (Appendix B)  307
Partial Pressure of a Dry Gas    198
Partial Pressure (in mm Hg) of Gases in the Air, Alveoli, and Blood (Appendix A)    307
$PCO_2$ to $H_2CO_3$    200
Periodic Chart of Elements (Appendix H)    313
pH (Henderson-Hasselbalch)    202
Poiseuille's Law    205
Predicted $P_aO_2$ Based on Age    207
Pressure Conversions    299

Relative Humidity    209
Review of Basic Math Functions    3
Reynolds' Number    212

Shunt Equation ($Q_{sp}/\dot{Q}_T$): Classic Physiologic    214
Shunt Equation ($Q_{sp}/\dot{Q}_T$): Estimated    218
Shunt Equation: Modified    222
Spearman-Brown Formula    276
Statistics Terminology    263
Stroke Volume ($SV$) and Stroke Volume Index ($SVI$)    224
Stroke Work: Left Ventricular ($LVSW$) and Index ($LVSWI$)    227
Stroke Work: Right Ventricular ($RVSW$) and Index ($RVSWI$)    231
Symbols and Abbreviations    291

Temperature Conversion (°C to °F)    234
Temperature Conversion (°C to K)    236
Temperature Conversion (°F to °C)    238
Test Reliability    275
Tidal Volume Based on Flow and $I$ Time    240
Time Constant    242

Units of Measurement    297
Using the Logarithm Table (Appendix M)    316

Vascular Resistance: Pulmonary    244
Vascular Resistance: Systemic    247
Ventilator Rate Needed for a Desired $P_aCO_2$    250

Weaning Index: Rapid Shallow Breathing ($RSBWI$)    254
Weaning Index: Simplified ($SWI$)    257